# STEP INTO ACTION

## WORKING THE TWELVE STEPS OF SEXAHOLICS ANONYMOUS

Sexaholics Anonymous
International Central Office
PO Box 3565
Brentwood TN 37024-3565
USA

Phone: (615) 370-6062
Fax: (615) 370-0882
Toll Free: 1-866- 424-8777
Website: http://www.sa.org
E-mail: saico@sa.org

ISBN 978-9755986- 8-9

*Table of Contents*

## *Appendices*

1st Edition

# *Introduction*

Countless thousands of men and women suffer from addiction to sex and lust in its many forms and from the consequences of acting out their lust. It is our hope that this book will bring understanding and encouragement to those whose actions are out of control. They are enduring great pain, shame, and guilt and seem to be powerless to change.

We are men and women who have suffered from sexual addiction and obsession with lust. We came to the rooms of SA where we learned that we no longer have to live that way. By working the Twelve Steps with a sponsor, within the fellowship of Sexaholics Anonymous, we found a better life, the gift of peace, freedom, happiness, and serenity.

We are forever indebted to the pioneers of Alcoholics Anonymous for their wisdom, insight, and perseverance. They provided the foundation upon which every Twelve Step recovery program is built.

We are grateful to our founder, without whose spiritual quest and determination, there would be no SA.

We thank all of our members who have traveled through their own personal hell to a life of sobriety, recovery, and gratitude. Their shared courage, strength, and experience made this book possible. We have been blessed beyond measure by the God of our own understanding. Ours has been a spiritual journey, from death to life, darkness to light, sickness to recovery.

We hope that you will join us.

# *Foreword*

The idea of creating a Twelve Steps for SA has been around probably as long as our Fellowship itself. Step into Action covers the Twelve Steps of SA's Twelve Step Program. The idea gained Fellowship-wide recognition during the emergence of the evolving service structure in the mid-1990s. In January 2000, the Trustees authorized the creation of a *Twelve and Twelve for SA*; in September of that year, a joint conference of Delegates and Trustees tasked the Literature Committee with bringing this project to fruition. Soon thereafter, work began on collecting material for the book. At a Fellowship workshop in Chicago in April 2004, a basic outline for the book was adopted. In addition to practical guidance for working each Step, the book would include a "Tools Section," "Member Shares," and "Recommended Readings" from Fellowship approved literature. The new SA Twelve Step book would be written by SA members for SA members. The Trustees approved the outline for the new book in July 2004, and the first volume of the Step into Action series, *One, Two, Three* became available a year later. The second book *Four, Five, Six, Seven* was published in April 2007; and the third and final book of the series, *Eight, Nine, Ten, Eleven, Twelve* was published in November 2008.

All of the *Step into Action* volumes were ascribed "work in progress" status, meaning they would be accepted as Fellowship approved literature subject to updates and incorporation of feedback before the final combined edition was submitted to the General Delegate Assembly again for approval. The books were—and continue to be—used by individuals and by groups, working alone and with sponsors, at Step workshops, on the phone, by Internet video chat, and email. Since their initial publication, all volumes have had multiple printings. With each release, feedback was solicited, and voluminous feedback was received.

The decision to combine all Twelve Steps into one volume was made by the Board of Trustees at the SA Convention in Baltimore, in July 2013. Thus began the task of collecting and sorting feedback submitted over the years by individuals and groups, as well as creating new material found lacking in the original volumes.

One advantage the newly-appointed editors enjoyed over their predecessors was the availability of years of thoughtful feedback not available to the original editors.

It is not possible to list all individuals or groups that contributed to this volume, or to adequately express our gratitude for their valuable contributions. We also express our deep appreciation for the many editorial hours dedicated to selecting, editing, and formatting submissions. This book is offered in a spirit of humility as suggested guidance to those working the Twelve Steps of Sexaholics Anonymous. This *Step into Action* book reflects the collective experience, strength and hope of the SA Fellowship in working the Steps, and has been approved by the group conscience for use by all.

Thus the end of one long and painstaking process marks the beginning of another—or at least a significant milestone in its continuation—of our common journey through the Steps. Our prayer is that this guide will be used to work the Steps, and that the lives of its readers may be blessed, and they in turn prove to be a blessing to others.

## *The SA Sobriety Definition*

> *The only requirement for membership in SA is a desire to stop lusting and become sexually sober. In defining sobriety, we do not speak for those outside of Sexaholics Anonymous. We can only speak for ourselves. Thus, for the married sexaholic, sexual sobriety means having no form of sex with self or with persons other than the spouse. For the unmarried sexaholic, sexual sobriety means freedom from sex of any kind. And for all of us, single and married alike, sexual sobriety also includes progressive victory over lust. In SA's sobriety definition, the term "spouse" refers to one's partner in a marriage between a man and a woman (SA* 191-92*).*

Our fellowship-wide sobriety definition and our identification of lust as the core of our problem make Sexaholics Anonymous unique. The founding members of SA had tried other definitions of sobriety: sex only in "committed relationships;" masturbation as a "healthy outlet;" looking and fantasizing without acting out; anonymous sex so nobody gets hurt; and many others. These other definitions of sobriety may work for some who identify as sex addicts, but they did not work for those who called themselves sexaholics. It is important to note that these early SA members, who voted unanimously to adopt SA's sobriety definition represented all aspects of our addiction, including married, single, opposite-sex and same-sex attracted.

Although SA's sobriety definition has been consistent from the beginning, periodically throughout our history some individuals and groups have argued in favor of changing it. Instead of affiliating with an S-fellowship consistent with their personal philosophies, they attempted to change SA. Thankfully, our Tradition of placing principles before personalities (Tradition 12) and our Tradition of staying out of outside political and cultural issues (Tradition 10) have always prevailed.

Most SA members assume that our definition of sexual sobriety is understood and accepted by all who attend our meetings. Most groups read our sobriety definition at the beginning of every meeting. Many members who initially had reservations about our stand on sobriety found that—through working the SA program of recovery—they become able to accept our sobriety definition. Some, however, do not. We do not debate or seek to change anyone's mind; everyone has a right to their own beliefs. But we do encourage everyone to affiliate according to their own conscience and preference. SA is not for everyone who needs it; SA is for those who want it.

We have a solution. We don't claim that it's for everybody, but for us, it works. If you identify with us and think you may share our problem, we'd like to share our solution with you.

We have discovered, sometimes at great personal cost, that our personal recoveries depend on SA unity (Tradition 1), and we want to make sure everyone understands SA's position on sexual sobriety. For us, this is a matter of life and death. For us, SA sobriety works. We believe it can also work for you.

## *Practical Suggestions for Using This Book*

This book is a practical guide to working the Twelve Steps of Sexaholics Anonymous. It is intended as a resource for sexaholics who are working the Steps with a sponsor.

1. Each Step in this book begins with a section that explains the Step from the SA perspective. This is not meant to be the final word on the subject. Instead, the text is intended to serve as a springboard for further questions, deliberation, meditation, and study primarily by a sponsor and sponsee, and also by SA groups and individuals who have already worked through the Steps with a sponsor.

2. In each Step, the next section is Members of SA Share. These short stories offer a glimpse into how various members experienced that Step. These valuable observations and insights provide hope and inspiration as we work the Step and meet some of the same obstacles and struggles that were experienced by those who have gone before us.

3. The next section is Step into Action, the "how to" part. This section begins with Recommended Readings, which are listed in alphabetical order. These will help round out and enhance your understanding of the Step. We suggest that members read and study the Recommended Readings before working the Step.

4. After the recommended readings, One Method of Working the Step is described. This is not the only way to work that Step. The methods presented herein have been found to be effective for many members. But your sponsor's recommended way is the correct way!

5. The last section, Some Questions to Consider, is a list of questions related to the recovery principles covered by that Step. These are suitable as topics for meetings, for meditation or journaling, and for sponsors to use with sponsees in working the Twelve Steps. They can be answered orally or in writing.

# *Step One*

*We admitted we were powerless over lust—*
*that our lives had become unmanageable.*

Step One was a flat admission of defeat. "We are beaten," we said, "and we can't stop doing what makes us sick." Lust was killing us. There was an unexpected gift in this admission of weakness: by accepting reality, by acknowledging our disease, by embracing our failure, we found hope. This was the start of surrender. From the ruins of our lives, we began to build a road to recovery and health.

We started by looking at the words in the Step.

"We"—What did that mean? It's simple: "I" couldn't do this alone. "We" replaced "I." It was not enough for me to admit that I was a sexaholic. I had to admit it with you. I admitted it, you admitted it, we admitted it. When we admitted our powerlessness to others and they to us, something special happened. By admitting the truth about ourselves, the power the secret had over us somehow lessened. Some of the guilt and shame melted away and we began to look honestly at what was really going on in our lives.

What did we admit? We admitted that we were powerless. What does "powerless" mean? Here is the way one member described it:

> My car stops on the railroad track and will not start. I am locked inside. I cannot open the door. I cannot open the window. I cannot get out of the car. A train is coming. I am without power to stop the train from hitting my car, nor can I get out of the car to save myself. What is it that I am without power to do? That train rushing at me is lust. I am powerless over lust. Step One does not say that I am powerless over my compulsive sexual behaviors. I am powerless over lust.

What, then, is lust? Lust is excessive and unreasonable thoughts or feelings that drive us to use or manipulate ourselves, others, or things for self-centered destructive purposes. Lust is what we get when we impose a distorted spiritual attitude upon a natural drive. As sexaholics, we were obsessed with sexual lust. We were drawn helplessly to lust, repeatedly trading short-term pleasure for long-term pain. The more we acted out, the greater the lust hunger became; the greater the lust hunger became, the more we acted out. All of our efforts to control or stop lust were met with a reaction from the brain which now expected the stimulation provided by lust and experienced deprivation without it. Our compulsion to act on our lust deepened the obsession. We kept driving back onto the train track in spite of the growing awareness that we were in serious trouble.

We found that when we thought of something and kept repeating it in our heads, attaching a feeling to it, we eventually created it. In other words, a building is not created by putting bricks together; it is created from an idea of the architect who thought about it, dreamed about it, worked and labored to see it come to pass. When we permitted a lust thought to remain in our heads, we began physical, mental, spiritual, emotional, and neurological changes within us. If we repeated these lust thoughts, we often created the reality. Our creation—sex with self, or sex outside marriage, or some other form of destructive acting out—was the result of lust. Lust was more powerful than we were.

Awareness of our problem was fundamental to our attempt to obtain sobriety. One of the stumbling blocks in our efforts to become and remain sexually sober was our inability to fully understand, accept, and admit our powerlessness over lust. Our admission of powerlessness over lust was the way to physical, mental, and spiritual freedom. We learned that the essence of powerlessness for the sexaholic was—*we do something out of lust, we get a negative result, and yet we do it again in the vain hope of a different outcome. Our lives become unmanageable.*

The second half of this Step referenced the unmanageability of our lives. What did "unmanageable" mean? There were negative consequences that resulted from our acting out, and from the way we lived our lives to support our sexaholism. A list of examples of this unmanageability is almost as long as the number of SA members, but includes:

- We were often late for commitments or didn't show up at all because we were "busy".
- We lashed out in anger at loved ones (and total strangers) without control or remorse.
- We lost jobs or were arrested because of our behaviors.
- We remained distant from those around us because we were constantly thinking about our next "fix."
- Our computers were always full of viruses.
- We couldn't have healthy sex with our spouse because of the fantasies that played in our minds.
- We lost marriages or limped along in empty marriages.
- We lived in constant fear that our actions would be discovered, while simultaneously getting high from the rush of acting out.
- We could not complete tasks or meet our responsibilities because they conflicted with our need to feed the addiction.
- We lost friends or were unable to make friends.
- We avoided relationships and jobs because we were afraid.
- We wrecked careers, homes, and lives.
- We were hospitalized for depression or attempted suicide, because sexaholism destroyed our physical, emotional, and spiritual being.

Our inability to cope with life on life's terms accompanied our sexaholic thinking and behavior. We found that a life driven by lust brought with it confusion, chaos, misery, and disaster. We suffered in numerous ways and caused suffering for others, including those most dear to us. We disregarded our conscience and we invoked God's help while continuing the same sick behaviors. We experienced moral revulsion at doing that which we didn't want to do, but felt compelled to do nonetheless.

In Step One we admitted that we were powerless and that our lives had become unmanageable. We admitted it to ourselves, to our sponsor, and to our group. We broke out of our isolation. We finally exposed our secrets. We admitted defeat.

## *Members of SA Share*

*1*

For me it was simple. I had to be forced to admit defeat. Ego driven, I could not and would not admit failure. If I didn't admit that I was wrong, then I wasn't wrong. I would not give up. I would find a way. No matter what, I was not going to be defeated. My life was out of control, yet I knew I could make it work. I could make it different. I just needed another chance. Again and again I committed the same acts. Again and again I made the same promises to stop. No matter how hard I tried, I could not stop.

Totally out of control, I finally gave up. Lust had beaten me. I made a call and admitted that alone I could not stop. I needed help. I was lost inside myself and lonely. I had nowhere to go. Desperate, defeated in every way, I let go and came to SA. Only when I gave up could I hear others say, "Let go and let God." Then and only then did I accept that it was a "we" program. I never have to do it alone.

*2*

I found that trying to work this Step without a sponsor was pointless and hopeless. With my keen sexaholic mind, and since I had the "Twelve Instructions," I thought that if I just went to meetings, I could do this program by myself without a sponsor. I was willing to rely on the group for support, fellowship, and a place to dump my emotional garbage. I forgot that it was my best thinking that got me into the mess that I called my life. Continuing to relapse, I was unable to maintain sobriety until I was willing to begin to trust another member enough to ask him to be my sponsor and to listen to his instructions and his feedback about my Step work. I eventually trusted him with all my secrets. My sponsor helped me to see that working the first four Steps by myself was only an incomplete Step One. By following his directions completely, I stopped relapsing and strung together the first sexually sober period of my adult life.

I rewrote my First Step with my sponsor's guidance. This time I chose to give away my Step One inventory to my home group. For me, the acceptance from the group and the lack of condemnation and punishment, even when knowing my darkest secrets, was the closest thing I had experienced to unconditional love. I felt a true freedom for having given my Step One inventory away.

*3*

Our family had recently moved to a new city. My wife was pregnant with our second child. I had engaged in compulsive sexual behaviors for twenty-eight years. Slowly but surely lust had increased its stranglehold on my life. Once again I hoped that a change of location and career might stop my acting out, only to find it was increasing in frequency and severity. There was so little time in the day to act out that I began to get up in the middle of the night to go through my rituals—while the family slept. A new boundary crossed.

I was spending increasing amounts of time during the day fantasizing about what I was going to do that night. My lustful thoughts were turning increasingly dark and destructive. I had the definite feeling I would not live to see my wife give birth. My life looked great to most people. No one would have guessed how unmanageable it really was. I was working very hard to keep that fact hidden from everyone, especially myself. In fact, I was leading a dual life that was putting everything I cherished in danger.

My obsession with lust had led to my crossing one boundary after another. For example, I'd promised myself I would never act out at work. Yet that's precisely what I did, and had been doing for months, since being promoted. My boss had even walked into a room adjacent to the one where I was acting out and called my name. A few more steps and I would have lost my job and faced legal consequences and public exposure. I would have been separated from the family I loved.

Reading *Sexaholics Anonymous* helped me see that I was a sexaholic and could not stay sober by myself. SA helped me understand that lust was the driving force behind all of my acting out, and progressive victory over lust was the only way to freedom. I had been trying to stop my compulsive behaviors, but they were only symptoms of my real problem—lust!

The books of the SA Fellowship, *Alcoholics Anonymous, Twelve Steps and Twelve Traditions,* and *Sexaholics Anonymous* made it clear to me that I must begin my recovery by accepting my "devastating weakness and all its consequences." It helped me see that if I took hold of the program of Sexaholics Anonymous as a drowning person seizes a "life preserver," I could get well.

*4*

Coming into the Program, my powerlessness and unmanageability extended well beyond my lusting and acting out. I was powerless over my political and religious beliefs, and this almost kept me from finding recovery. I was offended by parts of SA's sobriety definition. I wanted a kinder, gentler, more enlightened form of sobriety. This fellowship was clearly wrong, and I intended to convince everyone of that fact!

My sponsor suggested that I set aside my crusade for the moment and focus on getting sober and starting my recovery. He pointed out that my ongoing, negative emotional focus on these issues made my recovery unmanageable. He said that after I was sober for a year, he would be willing to argue with me about this topic, if I really wanted to.

Now, after years of sobriety and recovery, I find I never did have that argument with my sponsor. I am grateful for SA and its sobriety definition.

*5*

Long before I had a name for my problem—sexaholism—I knew I was powerless over it. I had tried to stop countless times and failed every time. Over the years I had just come to accept this dark secret as a part of my life.

Finding out about SA gave me a sense of hope. At my first SA meeting I immediately related to people sharing about personal powerlessness over lust and sexual acting out. They told me that only a Power greater than themselves could relieve that lust. However, I did not understand their explanation about how their lives had become unmanageable. Even when I did my First Step at four months' sobriety, I still had not connected with my personal unmanageability.

Three months later, I sat in a treatment center for sexual addiction. I told my counselor that I understood the powerlessness part of Step One, but that I just did not see my unmanageability. In her very quiet and calm voice she pointed out the obvious: "For one, you are sitting here in a psychiatric facility for a thirty-five day treatment that is going to cost you about $20,000. That seems a little unmanageable." I reluctantly had to agree, but I went on to say, "Well, other than that I don't see any unmanageability." She replied, "Well, you are not working for these five weeks, you are eight hundred miles away from your wife . . ." Her listing the facts helped break through my denial. I compiled a list of over thirty incidents in which sexaholism had made my life unmanageable. The full weight of the devastation of my disease was overwhelming.

As my sobriety has grown through years of working the SA Program, I have become aware of even more ways in which my life had become unmanageable because of sexaholism. It is truly baffling to me that I could not see it clearly until I had been in recovery for some time. In retrospect, I see I did not really want to admit I was as sick as everyone else in those SA meetings. My disease wanted me to believe that somehow I was different.

The good news today is that I do not have to live with all of that unmanageability in my life. My life in recovery is proof that I have serenity and sobriety as long as I work the Steps and Traditions in all parts of my life, go to meetings, call my sponsor regularly, follow his directions, and let God lead my life.

*6*

The lesson of Powerlessness was easy to accept when I was in the despair of relapse. But once I got a little bit of sobriety, it was easy to forget powerlessness, and think that now I had gained some power. The real lesson of powerlessness for me was only learned through repeated relapse. In sobriety, and even in recovery, I remain powerless. I never gain power over lust, and I never will. Until I accept that I *am* powerless over lust, not that I used to be powerless over lust, I do not sufficiently surrender the little drinks and temptations of everyday life to my Higher Power. And it is only through total surrender that I become free.

*7*

Early in recovery, I associated unmanageability with the consequences of my disease. I had lost several marriages. Relationships had suffered. My employment had suffered. These consequences were real and were pointed out by my sponsor when I did my First Step. This view of unmanageability was helpful. Now, with a little bit of recovery under my belt, I'm coming to realize that the thought that I am competent on my own, that I can rely only on my own resources to manage my life is a lie. I need God's help and I need the advice and support of my recovery fellowship to navigate the twists and turns that life presents to me. It was pride that caused me to believe that I could manage my own life without assistance. I now consider it a sign of strength when I have the courage to ask for help.

*8*

I tried everything imaginable to stop my acting out. I tried prayer, Bible reading, and finding accountability partners. I cancelled my cable TV and Internet access at home. I promised myself that when my son was born I would stop. I said the same thing when my daughter was born. I disclosed my first affair to my wife and family and even considered tattooing a religious symbol on my private parts. In reality I could not stop and nothing in my power would ever be able to stop me. Lust was my answer to life's problems, and I needed a power greater than myself to help me. Thankfully I found that power in SA.

*9*

I had been practicing my addiction for over five decades, but it took the Internet to move it into hyper speed. It was there 24/7, and it was free. It controlled my everyday work life. I would arrive at work and do the things I needed to complete for the day and get on the Internet as soon as possible. The quicker I got my work done, the sooner I could get my fix. I thought surfing the Net was fun, but it had become my priority, my master, my life.

One day, I was invited to a meeting after lunch. I was told I could resign or be fired. There had been a system changeover and they found all the places I had been visiting on the Internet. I was caught. The day I had feared as the end of my life had arrived. I always thought I was too smart to get caught.

For the first time in my life, there was no way out—life was unmanageable. I couldn't even lie my way out. I had to go home and explain to my wife why I would not be able to return to work.

Instead of feeling total despair, I was at ease. It was as if a heavy load had been lifted from my shoulders. For the first time I was totally honest. People had seen who I was. I came to understand that instead of being the worst day of my life, it had actually been the best day of my new life.

### *10*

In 1987, my wife brought the White Book (*Sexaholics Anonymous*) home from a visit with a client. I had been sober for three years—an incredible gift of God, looking back at my life as it had been in my previous marriage. For three years, God had showered His love upon me and kept me free from acting out with prostitutes, at massage parlors, and with affair partners. But I had no idea of the disease concept. I just experienced myself having lived immorally.

The White Book gave me another incredible gift—insight into my real problem, lust. This drew me into the Program. The White Book suggested that getting sober was one thing, but our real goal is *recovery*. For that, I needed a program of daily work, and this is what SA gave to me. But after five years of Program and meetings, I felt unsatisfied with the constant "lust struggle." What I wanted was real freedom, and I conceived this as freedom not from lust, but from temptation to lust. I wanted to get rid of lust once and for all. So, I changed my sobriety definition to include immediate, total and complete surrender when tempted.

I was never able to live up to my new definition for very long, because I rarely believed that I had surrendered that image or that fantasy thought quickly and completely enough. The result was that I had to give up all my service positions because I could not stay sober to this new definition for even 30 days. And I couldn't find a sponsor who would work with me using my new definition.

This went on for a year or so, until I came to understand that I was on the wrong track, a track of arrogance. I tried to be stronger than Lust–to throw it out from me totally. And this turned out to be impossible. In fact, although I remained sober by SA's definition, I fell into great resentment that I couldn't stay sober by my definition. "Sobriety by works of the Law" did not work for me.

Finally, I surrendered. As the White Book says, "the realization slowly dawn[ed] that we may always be subject to temptation and powerless over lust. We come to see that it's alright to be tempted and feel absolutely powerless over it, *as long as we can get the power to overcome*. The fear of our vulnerability gradually diminishes as we stay sober and work the Steps. We can look forward to the time when the obsession—not temptations—will be gone" (*SA* 68-9). I returned to our common sobriety definition. I recognized the wisdom of "progressive victory over lust" and have been gratefully recovering ever since.

## *Step into Action*

### *Recommended Readings*

We suggest that members read and study the following before working the Step:

*Alcoholics Anonymous* (*AA*)
"The Doctor's Opinion" xxv-xxii
*"Bills Story"* 1 - 8
*"There is a Solution"* Ch.2
*"More about Alcoholism"* Ch3.

*Sexaholics Anonymous* (*SA*)
"The Problem" 26 - 59
*"Surrender – Steps One, Two, and Three"* 79 - 81
*"Step One"* 83 - 88

*Twelve Steps and Twelve Traditions* (*12&12*)
"Step One" 21 - 24

## *One Method of Working Step One*

### *A Personal Step One*

Many of us find that working a personal Step One with our sponsors is an excellent way to launch our Step work. We can take key words from the text of Step One and write out the meaning for each of those words. Then we sit down with our sponsor to look over the results of the assignment—a sheet full of definitions—and discuss the ones that seemed most applicable. Our list may look something like this:

> *Admit:* to concede, to acknowledge, to confess
>
> *Powerless:* helpless, incapable, unable, impotent
>
> *Unmanageable:* uncontrollable
>
> *Our lives:* our behaviors, actions, experiences

We write a short list of the acting out behaviors or triggers that brought us to SA. Our list might include: masturbation, internet chat rooms, internet images, objectification of others, pornographic images and videos, romantic fantasy, and prostitutes. Using all this information, we write out our own version of Step One:

> "I concede that I am completely incapable of handling lust, as it leads to my compulsive use of masturbation, internet images, chat rooms, objectification, pornography, fantasy and prostitutes—that I have lost control over my thoughts, feelings and actions."

We may write our personal Step One on a small card and carry it with us as a daily reminder of why we are members of SA. Next, we begin writing our First Step inventory.

### *Preparing a Written First Step Inventory*

When we arrive at Sexaholics Anonymous, we are told to go to as many meetings as possible, to get phone numbers of fellow members and start using them daily, to begin daily readings of the literature, and to get a sponsor (even if only a "temporary" sponsor) so that we can start working the Steps. We need a sponsor because deceit and lying has become so much a part of us that we often believe our own lies. In our denial, we continue our sexaholic thinking and behaviors. A sponsor helps shed light on our true condition.

We are also told that we need to write out our First Step with the help of our sponsor. The purpose of a written First Step Inventory is to come to know within ourselves that we really are sexaholics, that we are powerless over lust, and that our lives will remain unmanageable by us, if we don't find recovery.

This Step often brings up uncomfortable feelings as we see the written truth before us. Some of us spend afternoons at our sponsors' homes writing this list. Just having someone close by can provide a sense of safety from lust that allows us to face the pain, fear, and shame. Others write inventories at workshops where groups of recovering persons meet and support each other as they write about some really painful experiences. These gatherings allow us to do together what we cannot do alone.

Our sponsors caution us not to be surprised if some of this work arouses or triggers our lust, since lust may be our reaction to almost any strong emotion or situation. When this happens, we immediately make a phone call to our sponsor or another member of the Fellowship.

Once we finish writing our First Step Inventory, we meet with our sponsor to review it. Our sponsor points out any items we may have included for shock value or victimization rather than seeing our powerlessness and unmanageability. Our sponsor helps us word the examples in a way that tells the truth, without embellishment or drama, and that respects the feelings of the group members who will hear us present our Step One. We avoid specific details that might create triggers or legal problems for ourselves or for the members of the group.

Describing explicit, graphic images during the presentation of a First Step Inventory at an SA meeting is not appropriate. While "giving away" powerful images is sometimes needed in order to dispel their power, this is better done in private with a sponsor or another experienced SA member. In consideration of other group members, we do not use offensive language when giving our First Step.

The idea of telling our shameful secrets to our SA group does not appeal to many of us, but it is highly recommended. We call this "giving away" our First Step. In the early days of SA, few members had enough sobriety to act as sponsors, so this group sponsorship approach was developed. Each member presented their First Step to the group. This process led to group unity and helped each member begin to feel "part of" the Fellowship.

The taking of this Step can be scary. In the families and neighborhoods that some of us grew up in, revealing a weakness is like bleeding in front of a school of sharks. Some of us are also afraid that after we share the violent, abusive, and shameful nature of our acting out, other members will react negatively, with anger or disgust. Maybe we will be asked to leave! However, the response of the group is always otherwise; instead of condemnation, we receive love, acceptance, and support.

In this Fellowship, we speak of leading with our weakness. Presenting our First Step, admitting our powerlessness, is our first opportunity to do this. Understanding and accepting our powerlessness is our way to freedom.

In writing our First Step Inventory, we are careful not to focus on composing a great work of literature; we let go of all concerns about how good our writing looks or sounds. We scribble down the truth as it comes to us. Some sponsors ask us to simply create a chronological bullet list of incidences, rather than writing a narrative. Then, when we present our First Step, we share what happened in whatever words come to us. The focus is on where the disease took us—our powerlessness and the unmanageability of our lives—not on our eloquent writing skills. A bullet list also helps keep us from choosing just the right words that make us look more innocent than we really are.

Other sponsors may prefer that we write out our entire First Step in complete sentences as a narrative. That method is helpful for those of us who may be prone to getting off track when we speak, or those of us who may experience very strong emotions and would have difficulty articulating our thoughts in front of others.

In our First Step, we do not dwell on whose fault it is. The facts of our lives are just that—facts. It is not the purpose of this Step to judge where we, our parents, or anyone else has been right or wrong. The purpose is to admit to ourselves honestly that we are powerless and that our lives are unmanageable by us alone. The following are just a few of the questions we can consider in order to get started; most of us can easily add more questions with the prompting of our sponsor.

We start by looking at our sexual history. We think about our behavior, how we felt about it then, and how we feel about it now. We answer questions like these:

## *Some Questions to Consider*

1. What is my earliest recollection of sex? Was there anything compulsive or deviant about it?
2. Did I have any unusual pre-puberty experiences with sexual behavior?
3. When did I discover masturbation? Did it become compulsive and frequent?
4. What about visualization and romantic or sexual fantasy? Have these occupied a lot of my time?
5. Do I dress to attract attention?
6. Have I felt I had to have a relationship in order to feel okay about myself?
7. Did I engage in serial or overlapping relationships or affairs?
8. Did I use a sexual or romantic high to mask feelings?
9. Was the anticipation or the pursuit more important than the relationship? Did acting out ever really take away my craving for "more"?

10. Have I harmed myself or others physically, emotionally, or spiritually?
11. Have I experienced remorse, guilt, shame or depression because of my fantasies or behavior? Did my behavior conflict with my religious teachings or beliefs?
12. What finally brought me to SA? What were the final incidents?

Next, we think about powerlessness; that is, our constant vain attempts to control or stop lusting. We ask ourselves questions like these:

1. Were there times when I've been so consumed with lust that I was no longer aware of the world around me or able to think about the choices I was making?
2. Did I go to absurd lengths to be with my pornography, my romantic novel, or my current "relationship?"
3. Did I masturbate while driving? Did I act out sexually in public?
4. Did I have sex with persons who meant nothing to me or persons I didn't like? Did I objectify people? Did I notice only the attractive people in my environment?
5. What have I done that I didn't want to do? Whom have I associated with that I wouldn't have otherwise? Where have I gone that I otherwise never would have gone? Is lust running my life?
6. Did I do things that my better nature told me I shouldn't be doing? Did I put myself in dangerous situations in the pursuit of sex or lust?
7. Did I dress, flirt, or manipulate others in order to be lusted after?
8. Were there particular neighborhoods I could not drive through without acting out? Did I go to particular neighborhoods or places in order to stalk or spy on someone? Did I find myself looking in windows?

9. Did I do things that disgusted and overwhelmed me with shame?
10. Did I cross boundaries of behavior that I had set for myself? Was it impossible for me to say no?
11. What promises did I make to myself or to others? Did I keep them?
12. How many times have I tried unsuccessfully to quit? What happened when I failed?

Then, we list examples of the unmanageability in our lives, that is, the consequences of our addiction. Sometimes we can identify a direct consequence of an episode on the "powerless" list and place it on the "unmanageability" list. Examples of questions to guide our reflections are:

1. How much time have I spent in sexual obsession? How has time spent on the addiction affected other areas of my life?
2. How has my illness affected my home life, my spouse(s) (or lack of spouse), my children (or lack of children)?
3. What other relationships have been damaged by my acting out or obsession? What friendships have I lost?
4. Did lust interfere with a precious relationship, whether or not that person was the object of lust?
5. How has my illness affected my education or other areas of personal or skill development?
6. How has my illness affected my work, my career, or a promotion? Could I have been fired if discovered? Was I fired?
7. How has my illness affected my finances? Have I lost income or incurred significant costs? Have I remained trapped in an underpaid position because of my addiction?
8. Did I miss important events so I could act out? Did I create events, trips, or situations so I could act out?

9. How has my illness affected my reputation, my social standing? Have I or my loved ones received negative publicity or been under public scrutiny because of my acting out? Has it affected me legally?
10. Have I paid for or had an abortion to cover up my acting out?
11. Have I contracted or passed on a sexually transmitted disease?
12. Have I ever been arrested in my pursuit of sex or lust? Could I have been arrested for what I have done? Could I have been sued?

If we think that we can recover without the support of the group, some of us may refuse (or at least delay) giving away our First Step. However, our fear of returning to our addiction is usually greater than our fear of how the group might react. The support and acceptance we receive as we share our First Step breaks through much of the fear and shame we are carrying. We begin to see that we are no longer alone, that we have found a group of people who understand our problem and welcome us. A measure of relief from shame, fear, and isolation is one of the benefits of the First Step. Another is that if we are thorough in this effort, we have written evidence of the nature and severity of our condition. We begin to see the truth about ourselves and our addiction.

## *Step Two*

*Came to believe that a Power greater than ourselves could restore us to sanity.*

Step One helped us understand our predicament: our obsession with lust drove our thinking, always leading to progressively worse acting-out behaviors. We tried to stop and couldn't stop; we tried to moderate and couldn't moderate. Our insanity manifested in that inevitable instant where we once again believed that—this time—we could control and enjoy it. We were absolutely powerless over lust and the devastation it caused in our lives. And yet, we still wanted more.

Step Two showed us that there was a way out, and that we could get there if we followed others who had travelled the same road. One major gift of Step Two was hope.

Step Two promised that a source of power outside ourselves could give us relief from our sexaholism. We had become convinced that lust was more powerful than we were, but in SA meetings, recovering sexaholics spoke of a Higher Power who was restoring them to sanity—a Power greater than lust!

To begin with, that's all we needed to know. We were not asked to believe in someone else's idea of God. We were assured that SA is a spiritual program, not a religion. Steps Three and Eleven teach us that each member's Higher Power is the God of his or her own understanding.

It was certainly true that we came in with a great diversity of ideas and attitudes about God—the disease of sexaholism does not discriminate on the basis of creed or denomination! Many of us arrived with half-formed or muddled ideas about a Higher Power, and others had no meaningful concept of God at all. Some of us were agnostic and were not sure that God existed. Others were atheists, certain there could be no Higher Power presiding over the chaos that seemed to envelop our universe. Some thought there might be a Supreme Being, but did not believe that such a Being could or would solve their problems. Others among us had once believed in a personal God or had belonged to an established religion, but had lost faith and felt we were cut off from grace. Still others believed in God and participated in a faith community, but continued to struggle in the addiction's stranglehold. What did we have in common? We saw that we could not save ourselves. If we were to escape our bondage, we required more power than we alone possessed.

Our dilemma was whether we would choose to continue in the misery of our sexaholism, or whether we would be willing to explore the idea of spiritual help. There seemed to be no third option. The book *Alcoholics Anonymous*, the original Twelve-Step text, showed us the way out: "We found that as soon as we were able to lay aside prejudice and express even a willingness to believe in a Power greater than ourselves, we commenced to get results" (*AA* 46). We needed willingness and an open mind.

Many of us who had difficulty identifying a Higher Power began by thinking of the SA group as a "Power greater than ourselves." After all, here were people who suffered from the same disease as we did and who had found a way to overcome their problem. Surely this was more than we had been able to accomplish for ourselves. As we attended meetings, got to know other members, and heard others speak of the strength they drew from their Higher Power, we came to believe that there might be a Solution for our problem. The key was honesty, open-mindedness, and willingness. Attending meetings and connecting with sober members, we began to believe that a Power outside ourselves could relieve the mental obsession that afflicted us. We began to rely on that Power, asking for help in moments of powerlessness. We found that we could maintain sobriety one day at a time, one hour at a time, or even one temptation at a time. Some of us had prayed for relief from our sexual impulses and obsessions before; but having now experienced the support of SA meetings and this Fellowship, we felt a greater confidence in prayer. We felt a connection with our God.

As if the idea of a Higher Power wasn't enough of a challenge for some of us, we also found that Step Two contained a suggestion of insanity. If we need to be restored to sanity, then we must be insane! Some of us balked at this implication. Maybe we were willing to admit that we were sexaholic, but we did not consider ourselves insane. Perhaps, we had told ourselves, our actions while under the influence of lust demonstrated nothing worse than bad judgment or inappropriateness. This was where we once again had to take an honest look at the consequences of our acting out behaviors.

We again considered our Step One inventory. We found that we could identify the patterns of insane thoughts and actions towards people, places, and things that had wrought havoc in our lives and the lives of others. As we reviewed our inventory, we asked ourselves, "What sane person would repeat these actions that produced such pain, misery, shame, and loss?" In SA, we were told that repeating the same behaviors and expecting different results was in itself a definition of insanity. For most of us, the conclusion was clear: we were insane, and we needed help to find our way out. If we still had difficulty with this proposition, we discussed it with our sponsor and other members of the program with long-term sobriety.

Being restored to sanity meant giving up our rationalizations that our lies and sexual acting out hurt no one. We began to accept the truth that sex or romance could not fill the hole in our souls. We recognized that the "next one" would not save us, but would yield the same results as the last one, or the last one hundred. We acknowledged that we were not all-knowing, all-powerful, all anything. Step One helped us see these truths about ourselves. Step Two was the point in our work where we saw that we needed help to relinquish our insane behaviors. As we attended meetings and worked the program, we experienced a growing trust in our sponsors, our fellow addicts in recovery, the Twelve-Step program, and eventually a Higher Power of our own understanding. Our thinking changed from 'I can't do this' to 'I can't do this alone'.

## *Members of SA Share*

### *1*

This was the answer! A Power greater than myself was going to heal me from this terrible affliction. As I read "The Problem," "The Solution," and the Twelve Steps for the first time in *Sexaholics Anonymous*, I knew that I had found the answer that I had been looking for. The concept of a Power greater than myself, the one I call God, had to be the solution. I had come to the end of myself. I cried tears of relief and identification. My spouse had moved out, my career was crumbling around me, and I could not stop lusting for any extended period of time. Somehow and some way God was going to lead me out of this mess.

While I had no way of knowing how winding and twisting the path would be, I went to a meeting. God sent me a sponsor from a different faith tradition. As we worked the Steps together, we were able to do so because each was taking guidance from the God of his own understanding.

*2*

My sponsor told me that my Higher Power was whatever I knelt down in front of. I had knelt down in front of my brain because that was what I believed had worked for such a long time. It had allowed me to look successful; it had gotten me out of scrapes; it had allowed me to manipulate any situation so that I could live with myself. I could think my way out of my emotions by telling myself that was not how I was supposed to feel or that was not what I was supposed to think. I could rationalize a situation so that I could cope. How do I know that this is what I believed in? Because this is what I went to when I had problems. I went to my house of worship—me. I was addicted to me.

Lust was another god I held on to. The electricity of lust could give me hope on a bad day. I came to rely on it. I held on to mental images of my next wife in case the current wife didn't work out. I desperately needed the approval of other people to fill that deep hole inside me. I was overly sensitive to other people's opinions of me. My problem was that I wanted a standing ovation for taking out the garbage. I had to be right. I couldn't say that I was wrong about almost everything in my life. If I admitted that, the very thing I believed in—me—would be annihilated.

I came to SA, began to read the literature daily, and attended several meetings a week. I got a sponsor and began to work the Steps under his direction. I didn't act out. I made lots of phone calls to fellow members. Something wonderful was happening to me and I was not the center of it. I was coming to believe that a power greater than myself could restore me to sanity. Step Two allowed me to close my eyes, take a deep breath, and fall into the arms of my Higher Power.

*3*

Before I came to SA, I knew my life was unmanageable by me. I was afraid to admit this to others because I was afraid there was no solution. But at my first meeting I saw the solution at work. Self-described sexaholics were living happy and productive lives free from lustful thinking and sexual acting out. The problem got me in the door; seeing the solution in action brought me back. The "Power greater than myself" initially was the group.

When I saw the power of lust in my life, it was easier for me to connect with the second part of Step Two—that I needed to be restored to sanity. The unmanageability of my life under the influence of lust was obvious. My pursuit of porn had become obsessive. Masturbation had become my standard response to every form of stress. I was emotionally immature. I got angry easily, didn't take kindly to criticism. Sober from alcohol, I could no longer blame substances for my insane thinking and behavior. I was causing pain to myself and others while under the influence of a drug that was self-generated. If that's not insanity, I don't know what is! The Step Two reading in the White Book advised me, as one who had had success in quitting another addiction, to start at the beginning, as though I'd never heard of the Steps. I followed this guidance. I was coming to believe.

*4*

I am so grateful for the miracle of recovery! When I feel powerless, Step Two tells me there is a Power outside myself, greater than myself, which is ready, willing, and able to give me a daily and hourly reprieve from my addiction. That One is God. I continue to wrestle with the unmanageability of my character defects, which include jealousy, anger, and laziness. When I surrender to Him each defect as it arises, He relieves me of its power over me. Eight years sober now, I still struggle against the old feeling that I am not a good person. God continues to show me that I am a good and caring person.

*5*

Perhaps the most powerful aspect of working Step Two was the suggestion that I compose a list of attributes that my new Higher Power was going to have. I started out with attributes, and over time, this morphed into a list of affirmations that I repeated. Later, I reworded the affirmations into a prayer addressed to my Higher Power, and have made some adjustments over the years. The prayer that I say on my knees every morning now, which is my Second Step prayer, currently goes, "God, I thank you for being patient and forgiving. I thank you for loving me just as I am, and teaching me to love and trust myself. I thank you for giving me my emotions and granting me joy."

*6*

As a life-long agnostic/atheist, I was terrified of Steps Two and Three. How was I going to find a Higher Power I could turn my life over to?

When I shared my First Step to my home group—32 members strong—I was trembling and fearful. I then listened with rapt attention as my brothers and sisters gave me the most loving and helpful feedback I had ever received. I can't adequately describe it, but I felt Higher Power fill up the room, embracing me, and connecting me to my group. This is how I came to believe. I know I am in a spiritually connected space when I receive the gift of a public First Step share and feel the Higher Power in the room.

*7*

I came into SA with what I thought was a strong faith in a God that I could trust. But, in hindsight, I didn't act as if I believed. I worried about everything and tried to control everything. It wasn't until I really saw the evidence of Step One that it became clear to me how I desperately needed the God of my childhood faith. This Step One evidence consisted of prolonged suffering, devastations, desperation, and an utter lack of trust in anyone, including myself. In this spiritual desolation, I began to find hope in the God that I always thought I believed in. I had no other option but to trust God, and my God had to be trustworthy. If I trusted me, I was sunk.

The God of my childhood is a God that:

- Loves me unconditionally
- Is always on my side
- Gives me whatever I need to overcome obstacles and grow
- Is blameless for pain, suffering, and evil
- Is omnipotent and will eventually reveal all mysteries

This God I can trust. I have to.

*8*

My spiritual awakening was a very, very gradual process. I first had to become open-minded, willing, and honest. I needed to start praying again and make phone calls. I needed to agree with SA's Sobriety Definition. I needed to come to meetings, get a sponsor, and work the Steps, work the Steps, work the Steps, work the Steps, work the Steps. I needed to take direction, be a part of, and take part in the blessing of the Seventh Tradition. I needed to serve by carrying the message of my recovery to others—partly as an act of gratitude for the person who freely gave me what they had been given. I needed to own the wreckage of my past and become willing to make amends. The phrase "I was wrong when I ______" became part of my vocabulary. I now have an ongoing conversation with my dearest Friend (HP).

I walked into the rooms a wreck, but over time, through many miracles, I now walk in the world with God and others. Impossible Joy. Awakened to His way of life.

*9*

"Do I now believe, or am I even willing to believe that there is a Power greater than myself?" (*AA* 47)

On the spiritual journey, Step Two was simple and succinct—an adequate transition from admitting personal powerlessness to deciding to rely on God's power. I didn't need any more than to state my willingness to believe in a Power greater than myself, and to consider what I would like that idea of God to be for me. Thus was my cornerstone fixed in place, and I went forward with my sponsor's guidance through the book *Alcoholics Anonymous*.

"So, practicing these Steps, we had a spiritual awakening about which finally there was no question" (*Twelve Steps & Twelve Traditions* 109).

My remaining Step work brought me into the conscious awareness of the presence of God. It is well I didn't need to "figure out the God thing" in Step Two, for nothing I could have figured out in my mind could have revealed God's true grace, mercy, love, and efficacy as I came to experience it. I made the reality of these spiritual principles a way of life.

When the power and presence of God became the most important fact of my life, then I was drawn to "…face the proposition that either God is everything or else he is nothing" (*AA* 93).

My choice is that God is everything. Now the fullness of spirituality is opened and nothing can close it to me, save my own illness. "Our ideas did not work. But the God idea did" (*AA* 52).

*10*

I need to constantly revisit my Second Step. I first worked my Second Step about four years ago. There was no lightning bolt. I only became willing to believe in a Higher Power. That willingness is sometimes all that I have to hold onto when times are dark, but He is always there.

I unknowingly blocked all knowledge of my Higher Power under layers and layers of pride, procrastination, self-reliance, and a multitude of lies I told myself and others. I did all of this in the hope of keeping my life together myself—trying to stay one step ahead of my fears and shame. Though some of the wreckage has been lifted, I continue to add new pieces.

Each piece of damage I have caused lays there waiting for me to pick it up. Sometimes the damage is resentment from a childhood trauma. Other times it is my anger towards the person driving aggressively in front of me. However, each time I identify one of those pieces of wreckage to remove, I follow the path the Steps teach me. It's not enough for me to just point at the junk and ask God to take it away. Each time I need to pause, pray, and acknowledge that a Power greater than myself is necessary to remove it, that removal of the wreckage is essential for my sanity, and that sometimes God wants me to pick it up and throw it out myself—instead of just doing the same thing and hoping for a different outcome. Sanity is the real objective for me. When I finally acknowledge that, I can be willing to surrender to God.

### *11*

What SA has shown me and what Step Two shows me is humility. Listening to the stories of other successful and sane people, I had to admit that I did need restoring to sanity. I came to believe that something was uniquely wrong with me. This lust addiction—in the midst of a successful life—had me licked and always was there bugging me. God had tried a few times to get me to open up and deal with it and be true to myself, but I resisted and made excuses, like "men don't talk about masturbation and lust and ongoing struggles with pornography." I needed to come a lot further and more personally in my belief system. This God went to the heart of the matter, the true insane area that didn't fit with the public reputation I had. Face it all, is what I heard, and let God begin to restore you to a more complete and abundant life.

Humility, honesty and willingness to grow in faith is what I lacked. I let go, let God have it all, said it out loud, and Step Two became real. No more fighting, just a lot of accepting. God does a lot better with my life than I did. And this new level of partnership and surrender is a much more effective way to deal with this sexual stuff and all the other stuff in my life.

### *12*

When I first asked a long-time member how to "take" Step Two, he responded simply: "You could begin by dropping that resentment you have against the Church." Initially I was offended that a relative stranger could have me so well pegged, but I knew he was right. I had a chip on my shoulder about religion. I was constantly pointing out what I considered to be the hypocrisy of people who professed to have turned their lives over to God. Confronted by this member, however, I wasn't inclined to argue since I knew he was speaking from his own experience, and in my best interest. A fellow addict, he wasn't asking me to look at something he didn't have to look at in himself. I took his direction. I didn't need much persuasion to let go of a burden I had carried around for years.

SA doesn't require that I believe in any particular concept of God. In fact, in SA I found people who measure spiritual progress as much in terms of how completely we can surrender old ideas about God as in forming new ones. I was free to let go of beliefs that held me in spiritual bondage and to practice principles that worked. "Why don't you choose your own conception of God?" the literature suggested (*AA* 12). Suppose God wasn't a czar of the Heavens, condemning me, but was a Friend who walked beside me, helping me? This was a beginning and a practical concept I could build on.

## *Step into Action*

### *Recommended Readings*

We suggest that members read and study the following before working the Step:

*Alcoholics Anonymous* (*AA*)
"Bill's Story" 8-16
"*We Agnostics*" Ch.4
"*Spiritual Experience*" Appendix II 567

*Sexaholics Anonymous* (*SA*)
"Step Two" 89-92
"*Overcoming Lust and Temptation*" 157 - 168

*Twelve Steps and Twelve Traditions* (*12&12*)
"Step Two" 25 - 33

## *One Method of Working Step Two*

Some of us don't want to work Step Two. For many reasons, we don't like the idea of God or even the concept of a Higher Power. But we can't argue the fact that lust is more powerful than we are. And if there is nothing more powerful than lust, then there is no hope for us. Others think that working Step Two is unnecessary––"I already believe!" But as the author of SA's White Book, used to say, "If you're a lustaholic like me, your relation with God is wrong, regardless of what your belief or religious experience is. How could it be right if you're thinking and doing the things you tell me you're thinking and doing? To recover, your relation with God must change." We all need to work this Step!

Many of us find that writing a Step Two inventory is helpful at this early stage of recovery. This inventory is meant to help us consider what wrong ideas we may have developed about our Higher Power from interactions with the people in our lives that had power or influence over us. Our relationships with these people may well have shaped our attitudes and concepts of higher powers – even if we don't realize it. Discussing this inventory with our sponsor helps us realize how past experiences may have planted some wrong ideas into our minds. These old ideas may need to be discarded and replaced before we will even consider surrendering to a Higher Power in Step Three.

### *A Step Two Inventory*

We open a spiral notebook so that there are two blank facing pages on which to write. We divide the left hand page into three columns. The right hand page is the fourth column. On the left hand page, we label the far left column (col.1), "Powerful People"; the middle column (col. 2), "What Happened"; and the right-hand column (col. 3), "What I Learned (Old Ideas)." We label the right hand page (col. 4), "The Truth I Choose to Believe Today."

We complete the columns in order, from top to bottom. In the first column (col. 1), "Powerful People," we begin by listing the people who had power over us throughout our lives. For most of us, Mom and Dad head the list. Other powerful people may include stepparents, grandparents, siblings, neighbors, teachers, religious figures, or even lawyers or district attorneys. In column 2, describe your experience with this person, and in column 3, - what -you came to believe about "a power greater than you." See the example below.

As we list our experiences, we begin to see some of our old ideas that may get in the way of working Step Three. Since we may not even be aware that we hold certain negative beliefs about higher powers, we find it helpful to consider what someone who has had to interact with the people in column 1 *may* have learned. While I might initially think that I don't hold to a specific negative idea, my sponsor can sometimes point out behaviors that indeed appear to demonstrate that I actually do believe them. We do not worry if some of the experiences and ideas seem repetitious; these may be the deeply ingrained beliefs that most need to change.

Once this portion of the inventory is completed, we have identified some ideas and false beliefs which may be keeping us from recovery. Some of us find the ideas presented in Chapter 4 of *Alcoholics Anonymous* to be helpful. We discuss these with our sponsors or with members of the clergy or some other spiritual guides.

In column 4, we write what we now choose to believe about our Higher Power. When we have completed this column, we have described some of the attributes of a Higher Power who can restore us to sanity. We distill these new ideas into a list of simple statements about our Higher Power that we can affirm every day. Again, we do this with a sponsor, clergy, or other spiritual guide. Write these affirmations down and make them a part of our morning prayers.

*Step Two Inventory Example*

| *Col. 1* | *Col. 2* |
|---|---|
| *Powerful People:* | *What happened:* |
| Mom | Beat me and my siblings for small or imagined mistakes |
| | Was paralyzed by fear when my sister was injured; could not even take her to the doctor |
| Dad | Was always at work; didn't have time for his children |
| | Did not protect me or the other kids from Mom. |
| | Made us go to church, but kept a secret stash of pornography; observed him staring at attractive women |
| Boss | Was constantly critical of my work; pointed out my mistakes in front of others |
| | Fired me first when layoffs began |
| District Attorney | Assumed the worst about me |
| | Continued digging for any possible way to charge me with a crime, even after the initial charges were dropped |

*Step Two Inventory Example*

| *Col. 3* | *Col. 4* |
|---|---|
| *What I learned: (Old Ideas)* | *Truth I choose to believe today:* |
| My Higher Power is cruel and will punish me harshly | My Higher Power is kind and loving; I am not punished *for* my sins, but *by* my sins when He is angry. |
| I can't count on a Higher Power; I must take care of myself. | My Higher Power knows my needs and provides for me. |
| God is too busy for me; He does not concern Himself with my daily activities | My Higher Power delights in me; When I turn to Him, He is always there for me. |
| My Higher Power doesn't care about my pain. | My Higher Power feels my pain; His love for me is unchanging and everlasting. |
| Lust is OK for people who follow the rituals that God requires of us. | Lust is an abandonment of God; It poisons me spiritually and separates me from Him. God offers me freedom from lust through a loving relationship with Him |
| My Higher Power is judging and condemning. | God forgives me and won't give up on me; He is always there to pick me back up again, as soon as I turn towards Him. |

| *What I learned (cont'd): (Old Ideas)* | *Truth I choose to believe today (cont'd):* |
|---|---|
| Any imperfection makes me worthless to God. | My imperfections and failures remind me of my need for a Higher Power and provide an opportunity to surrender them to Him. |
| God doesn't understand me; God doesn't want to understand me. | God knows the thoughts and intents of my heart; He knows what I am and what He intends me to be. |
| My Higher Power wants to find one speck of wrong in me and then condemn me to die. | My Higher Power works patiently with me to reveal the shortcomings that are blocking me from His love, so that I can surrender and be free (so I can live!). |

## *Some Questions to Consider*

1. What areas of insanity do I see in my life? Will I list them and share them with my sponsor?
2. What does sanity mean to me? How would I like to be different?
3. What boundaries have I crossed with acting out that I never intended to cross?
4. Whom do I hold responsible for my problems in life? Myself? God? Other people? Why?
5. Do I believe that self-knowledge will cure me? Explain.
6. Do I think that I am capable of ever restoring myself to sanity?
7. What is my understanding of a God of my understanding?
8. If I could design my own Higher Power, what would that Higher Power look like?
9. What new ideas about a Higher Power am I willing to consider?
10. What kind of spiritual experiences have I had?

## *Step Three*

*Made a decision to turn our will and our lives over to the care of God as we understood Him.*

Steps One, Two, and Three are the core of the admission, submission, and surrendering process. At first glance, Step Three appears to be the point when we completely turn over our will and our lives, but few of us were willing or able to surrender everything immediately, in one grand gesture. Step Three asks us to *make a decision* to turn our will and our lives over to a Power greater than ourselves. Carrying out this decision is a daily, life-long process. Essentially, when we took Step Three, we committed to stop living by self-will. Instead we sought guidance from a Higher Power. We did this one day at a time by working the Steps in a spirit of willingness and surrender.

Who is this Higher Power to whom we turned over our lives? In Step Two, we had begun to develop a personal, working definition of the God of our understanding. Step Three helped us to grow in understanding and trust. We began to approach, and connect with, a trustworthy and loving God to whom we could surrender our will and our lives.

Because we struggled with self-will, and because for most of us procrastination was easier than action, working with a sponsor relieved us of the burden of solitary, unaccountable decision making. It helped us get out of our own heads. After all, it was our best thinking that brought us to this place! In recovery, we saw that self-knowledge and intellect were overrated when it came to overcoming our addiction. A sponsor provided guidance, support, and accountability. Working with a sponsor helped us prepare ourselves for the rigorous honesty required by Step Four. By doing this work we demonstrated the early signs of willingness and, in some cases, an eagerness to do God's will, instead of trusting our own self-will. Thus began a change of attitude that fostered openness, promoted integrity, and allowed us to remain teachable.

Many of us began by making the decision to turn over one problem, one event at a time, just as we live our sobriety one day at a time. We made it a daily exercise in letting go and letting God. Sometimes this decision meant making a phone call, asking for guidance, praying, going to a meeting, doing the next right thing, or exercising restraint while waiting for stormy emotions to subside. As we experienced moments of peace that came with turning over a few problems, we gained confidence and faith. By asking for help from a Higher Power, we admitted that we could not do it alone and opened ourselves to a Power who could help. When we found ourselves taking back control, we immediately made the decision to surrender the lust thoughts, resentments, fears, or other character defects again and again.

When we were running the show, our thoughts were out of control and regularly turned to lustful fantasies. We were plagued by fear, anxiety, despair, resentment, and self-loathing. We imagined we had good spiritual intentions, but rarely took good spiritual action. Our choices created painful consequences, and many of our actions were a source of shame and revulsion. Our relationships with those closest to us were poisoned with bitterness and neglect. What did we have to lose by giving up self-will and turning our will and our lives over to a Power greater than ourselves? With this decision, we accepted God's help without reservation. Often, God's help came to us as our sponsor's guidance and suggestions. Step Three meant giving up control over outcomes and instead opening ourselves to God's will. It also meant trusting God's guidance in everything we did. When we followed through on this decision, we got power back; it was God's power, not ours, and it enabled good action as our power never could. When our will was aligned with God's will for us, our lives became richer and fuller than we could ever have imagined.

The first paragraph of page 63 in *Alcoholics Anonymous* describes the benefits we experienced when we turned our will over to God. Some refer to these as the "Third Step Promises."

> When we sincerely took such a position, all sorts of remarkable things followed. We had a new Employer. Being all powerful, He provided what we needed, if we kept close to Him and performed His work well. Established on such a footing

> we became less and less interested in ourselves, our little plans and designs. More and more we became interested in seeing what we could contribute to life. As we felt new power flow in, as we enjoyed peace of mind, as we discovered we could face life successfully, as we became conscious of His presence, we began to lose our fear of today, tomorrow or the hereafter. We were reborn.

Beyond our daily surrender to God, the decision to surrender our will and our lives was a decision to work the rest of the Steps. Step Three is a call to action. As *AA*'s *Twelve Steps & Twelve Traditions* puts it: "Like all the remaining Steps, Step Three requires action, for it is only by action that we can cut away the self-will which has always blocked the entry of God—or, if you like, a Higher Power—into our lives" (34). For us sexaholics, giving up self-will meant working the Steps, and the action of working the Steps gradually lifted the fog of self-obsession. God's power and love flowed into our lives, bringing with them a sense of inner peace.

> We were now at Step Three. Many of us said to our Maker, as we understand Him:
> God, I offer myself to thee—to build with me and to do with me as Thou wilt. Relieve me of the bondage of self, that I may better do Thy will. Take away my difficulties, that victory over them may bear witness to those I would help of Thy Power, Thy Love, and Thy Way of life. May I do Thy will always! (*AA* 63)

Peace was the direct result of a life where we did not have to be in charge anymore. Brooding, fretting, resenting, and lusting were replaced with the simple responsibility to seek, listen, and follow. To our surprise and delight we learned that daily surrender to a Higher Power not only relieved the tyranny of sexaholism, it manifested in all aspects of our lives. We saw improvement in our relationships, our work, our finances, and even our health. These were the natural consequences of placing our lives under better management. With gratitude, newfound optimism, and tangible success in our own program of recovery, we found ourselves ready to begin working on Step Four.

## *Members of SA Share*

*1*

When I first read Step Three in the White Book I thought it was the simplest of the Twelve. After all, it's only a "decision." I figured the Step would take me all of five minutes, mirroring the experience described in the personal story "Flooded with Feeling" (*AA* 369-374). When I said my "Third Step Prayer," however, nothing seemed to happen. My sponsor suggested that, just like making other significant life decisions, perhaps deciding to turn my will and life over to God's care is more of a process than a one-time event. I thought about what he said and endeavored to work Step Three until it took hold.

As I looked back, I saw that when I was finally serious about getting sober, I got a sponsor. Then I actually heeded my sponsor's advice. Those first acts of surrender were my first pieces of evidence that something truly supernatural was happening, because deference did not come naturally to someone as impressed with himself as I was.

I crossed another milestone on the Step Three journey when I set up renewal partners for each morning of the week. We committed to turning our will and the care of our lives over to God for the day. Over time I became close with most of my partners and developed a network of program friends with whom I could share anything.

*2*

To die a sexaholic death or to live life on a spiritual basis—both seemed hard choices. The decision to turn my life and my will over to my Higher Power was made easier by the evidence that my inability to run my life was killing me. I was relieved to hear that a Power greater than myself would do the job perfectly and that all I had to do was to act as if He was! I had to practice turning over my will. I practiced turning over my desire for a relationship and marriage, my terrible emptiness, my longing for old boyfriends, and my fears. Gradually, I found that the more I gave it over to Him, the easier my life became.

*3*

When I came to SA I was desperate. The affairs, the constant thoughts of sex, and the masturbation fantasies were out of control. As I listened to the Steps being read at meetings, however, I knew "God" was going to be a problem. I was a life-long atheist, but I realized that the first two Steps said nothing about God. I would get sober and deal with the "God" problem when I got to Step Three.

For the first year, I used other names for God. Master, Teacher, and Higher Power were acceptable. After sharing my Step One inventory with an SA group, I met with my sponsor to do the next two Steps—the two I most dreaded. He said he would have me do exactly what his sponsor did with him.

He asked, "Do you believe a Power greater than yourself can restore you to sanity?"

I said, "Yes."

He asked, "Are you willing to work Steps Four through Twelve?"

"Yes."

"Now you need to begin writing your Step Four inventory."

I was shocked. My readiness to fight "God" in Step Three was unnecessary. "The care of God *as we understood Him*" meant just that: as I understood Him. My sponsor said that he understood that the "decision to turn our will and our lives over" to God meant I was willing to no longer be in charge. I was willing to follow my sponsor's direction and work the rest of the Steps.

*4*

At one point as I was struggling with this Step, my sponsor suggested I go to a nearby thoroughfare, flag down the first car that would stop, and turn my life and will over to the care of whoever was driving. He asked me how they could possibly screw it up any worse than I had. Another old-timer said I could just as well pick someone sleeping on a park bench and let him be my Higher Power. I might see some improvement in my current circumstances. They were both right. My best thinking was self-will run riot.

*5*

In a hotel 800 miles from home, I was spending a weekend in service work with a small group of sober sexaholics. As we worked in a conference room near the elevator platform on our floor, we could see children running past our window and hear them call to each other. I touched the arm of a fellow member and asked him to step outside with me. There, leaning against a railing, I told him, "I need to check in."

"I'm very aware of these children around us today. I have children of my own and I respond to children, but I've also molested children. As far as I can tell, I'm not experiencing any sexual excitement, and I'm not struggling with the desire to lust. But that's what this energy I feel around me can turn into. So I want to turn it over to God before it gets to that point. With you as my witness, I'm acknowledging my powerlessness to God. I ask God to give me surrender over the desire to lust this morning. I believe that by opening myself up to you I open myself to God. I appreciate your listening."

I said that without pausing. We maintained eye contact the entire time. He thanked me for sharing, and we went back to work. I had no trouble that morning or for the remainder of the weekend.

That's one way I can turn my will and my life over to the care of God. When I affirm my powerlessness to another sexaholic, I'm giving it to God; I know I'm no longer alone with it.

*6*

The first time I read Step Three, it seemed a vague notion. However, I have found that I must be deliberate and specific about working the Steps, so I looked at the words carefully. Step Three did not say that my life and my will are turned over—it says I make a decision. What did that mean to me?

My life is influenced largely by the thoughts I entertain and the actions I take. Then, for me, my life is the sum of my actions.

The things that influence my actions are my thoughts. Step Three therefore required that I make a decision to turn my thoughts and my actions over to the care of God as I understood Him. This primarily means I make a decision to work the rest of the Steps.

*7*

I struggled with Step Three for a long time. My image of God was a cruel, indifferent Power who would punish me harshly whenever I angered Him. The decision to turn my will and my life over to Him came only after I had identified my false beliefs about God. The decision I made was to let go of those old ideas and identify the beliefs and ideas by which I was going to live my life from that moment forward. I realized that Step Three was a decision to continue an effort to develop a relationship with this Higher Power who could and would restore me to sanity if He were sought. I knew this was my last, best hope for freedom, and I pursued it. Today, as a result of this program, I know that I am the beloved child of a God who delights in me!

*8*

I believed that my Higher Power could restore me to sanity. I guess I always believed He *could*, but I wasn't sure that He *would*. I didn't feel I deserved it. I knew how I was supposed to act, but I still did bad things. I was active in church and thought I knew a lot about God, but I still acted out. I thought I deserved His judgment rather than His help. I was also afraid. My fear was that if I truly turned my life and will over to God and worked this program of recovery, I still might act out again. Then, I'd have tried everything and failed—there would be no hope left. While I still hadn't tried everything, there remained some slim hope. I now see that the Enemy (my addiction) was using this fear to keep me apart from God. Turning my life and will over to God isn't my last chance for recovery. It's my *only* chance for recovery! My sponsor helped me understand that God can not only help me gain lasting sobriety, He *wants* me to have lasting sobriety.

## *Step into Action*

### *Recommended Readings*

We suggest that members read and study the following before working the Step:

*Alcoholics Anonymous* (*AA*)
"How It Works" 60-63

*Sexaholics Anonymous* (*SA*)
"Step Three" 93-96

*Twelve Steps and Twelve Traditions* (*12&12*)
"Step Three" 34-41

## *One Method of Working Step Three*

An effective approach to working Step Three involves prayer, writing, and concrete action.

### *Prayer*

In addition to the Third Step Prayer, the "Submission Prayer" can be a source of inspiration:

> God, I give this day to you.
> Establish the work of my hands,
> the steps of my feet,
> the words of my mouth,
> the direction of my gaze,
> the thoughts of my mind,
> and the attitude of my heart.

We set aside some quiet time to pray. Many choose the morning, but others choose different times, such as at a meal or before retiring for the day. If a topic does not come to mind, we focus on a particular aspect of the two prayers, or express thanks to our Higher Power for the program of SA. We pray for the willingness to surrender doubt that this program will work.

### *Writing*

We often find it is helpful to write down the feelings and thoughts we have about working this Step. Am I looking forward to it or am I dreading it? What do we hope happens? What are we afraid might happen? Do we really want to turn our will over to God? Do we trust God enough to turn over our lives to His care?

In writing out responses to these questions, we find that some areas of life can be easily turned over to God's care. Other areas of life might be more difficult. This may be an indication that we need to do some more work on the earlier Steps. If we find it difficult to surrender because we feel that

God is not trustworthy or capable, we return to Step Two. When our ego will not relinquish certain aspects of life to God's care, we return to Step One. At the point where we have genuine willingness to "let go and let God," our prayers and writing will communicate that, and taking action will follow.

*Concrete action*

Actions speak louder than words. "Half measures availed us nothing" (*AA* 59). Here are some ways that we can take action with Step Three.

*Take direction from our sponsor.* As we work the Program, we soon realize we cannot profess to turn our will and life over to an Entity we cannot see or understand if we are unwilling to take direction from someone who has walked this path before us. That's not the way recovery works. Each of us—without exception—needs a sponsor. A sponsor usually has a greater degree of sanity, sobriety, peace, and wisdom than the sponsee. Working the program without a sponsor denies the principle of the Third Step. We demonstrate our sincerity and willingness to work this program of recovery by taking direction from a sponsor as we work the Steps. The "self-searching, the leveling of our pride" experienced in Step One helps make this possible (*AA* 25). We form a relationship with our sponsor, which means making a commitment to attending recovery meetings, working the Steps, and getting together regularly to review our Step work.

*Develop a network of program friends.* Early in recovery, some of us just want to get the meeting over with and get out of there. But we soon find that the friendly discourse among members—"the meeting before the meeting" and "the meeting after the meeting"—provides us an opportunity to ask for and receive feedback. We may have heard someone share during the meeting about an issue that we are experiencing. After the meeting, we can approach them, tell them our experience, and ask if they might share more about that topic. Over time our program friends grow close, and we find it easy to share anything with them. Along with our sponsors, this network of recovery partners creates the safe environment we need in order to learn and practice the principles of SA.

*The Third Step Prayer.* Some members in our Fellowship take this Step publicly by reciting the Third Step Prayer at meetings with other members joining in. Others may wish to do this with their sponsor or clergy.

> God, I offer myself to thee—to build with me and to do with me as Thou wilt. Relieve me of the bondage of self, that I may better do Thy will. Take away my difficulties, that victory over them may bear witness to those I would help of Thy Power, Thy Love, and Thy Way of life. May I do Thy will always! *(AA* 63*)*

*Use a Daily Renewal.* Many of us find a friend in the program to be an Accountability Partner or Daily Renewal Partner. We make contact with this person every morning and do a daily renewal to start our day. Here is one example of a daily renewal script, which participants ask each other in turn. *Practical Recovery Tools 1994 – 2003* has other examples.

1. Are you willing to admit you are powerless over lust?
2. Do you desire sobriety for the next 24 hours? (freedom from the obsessions and actions of lust, freedom from fear, resentment, shame, self-pity, etc.)
3. Are you willing to do whatever is necessary to protect this desire for the next 24 hours? (setting boundaries, prayer, reading, physical care of your body, reaching out and calling others)
4. Are you planning to do anything you would be ashamed of today?
5. Do you understand that at the end of this 24 hours you are free to choose this sobriety for another day or go another way?

6. Just for today, are you willing, with me, to hand over your will and your life to the care of the One who kept you sober yesterday and protected you from the full consequences of your lust in the past?
7. What are you grateful for today? (Gratitude is an antidote to lust.)

We keep it simple and brief. Our goal is just to remind ourselves that we are sexaholics, that we are sober, and that we wish to stay that way today.

## *Some Questions to Consider*

1. What decisions to change have I made that I would not have made when I first came into the program?

2. Am I willing to work with a sponsor on a regular basis? List how I do that.

3. Am I willing to follow my sponsor's suggestions?

4. What changes do I see in myself? In my daily life?

5. What thoughts, habits, and parts of my life do I still need to surrender?

6. Am I willing to turn my will and life over to a Power greater than myself? List those actions I am willing to take on a daily / hourly basis, one day at a time.

7. Am I willing to share these answers with my sponsor?

# *Step Four*

## *Made a searching and fearless moral inventory of ourselves*

Walking into our first meeting was intimidating, but soon attending meetings felt normal, helpful, and welcome. At meetings, we learned things we could not have learned in any other way. The Fourth Step was much like that. At first it looked intimidating; but like any other tool, once we learned how to use it, it became our friend. We were not in the habit of honestly looking at our own strengths, our weaknesses, or our problems relating with others. However, we were told that mastering the skill of accurate self-inventory is essential to recovery. Stamped into the anniversary tokens we receive in recognition of various lengths of successful sobriety is the admonition "To thine own self be true." So we moved forward. Delay or avoidance would leave our recovery on precarious footing. We needed to know the truth about ourselves. In Step Four, we began an extended exercise in honest self-discovery. This process of taking stock of our physical, emotional and spiritual selves was illuminating and liberating.

Whether or not we admitted it, we felt shame and fear about our character defects and guilt and remorse about our actions. We tried to escape from these dreadful feelings by lusting. Resentment, fear, and shame were triggers for our lust, often without our being aware of it, and lusting led to acting out. Each episode of acting out caused more self-loathing and the cycle got worse and worse. Step Four helped us find and admit the problems we needed to work on and needed help with. It helped us to get out of denial and to break the cycle. It gave us a tool to use on our resentment, fear, and shame *before* they triggered lust.

Our pursuit of the truth was to be *searching* and *fearless. Searching* meant that the inventory had to be methodical and thorough. We needed to be willing to expose and examine all aspects of our thinking and behavior, in all areas of our lives. A thorough inventory would include everything, good and bad. It was not enough to acknowledge our everyday shortcomings, to admit our more obvious acting-out behaviors, or to see our superficial abilities. We had to probe those basic character traits that got in the way of a full and productive life. We had to acknowledge those strengths and resources that had helped us survive and would assist in our recovery. We examined the inner structure of our character to discern what was sound and what might give way at any moment. We prayerfully followed our sponsor's directions and kept at the task.

*Fearless* meant that we were willing to face the truth about ourselves. It didn't mean that we were without fear. On the contrary, we were afraid but took the action anyway, supported by our faith. Our faith helped us to ask, "What is the worst that could happen if I do this?" Our Step work thus far helped us believe that the potential benefits of Step Four outweighed any risk. We were coming to believe that a benevolent Higher Power could manage our life better than we could. We had already made the decision to turn our thinking and behavior over to the God of our understanding, so it wasn't our place to be judgmental about ourselves anymore. We didn't use our fear as an excuse to delay. We found the courage to work Step Four.

If we were to have peace of mind, we first had to examine those elements of our thinking and feeling that drove our behavior. Like cleaning a closet, we attempted to rid ourselves of the things that were no longer of use to us. These might be survival instincts or coping mechanisms that had worn out their welcome. Now they caused more harm than good to ourselves or to others. They got in the way of our attempts to behave as responsible adults. Our Fourth Step inventory helped us to conclude that these attitudes and habits had become liabilities rather than assets.

Many of us were so overwhelmed by self-loathing that we were unable to see anything worthwhile in ourselves. This sort of negative pride impeded our growth and threatened our sobriety. Our fear told us that there would be nothing left if we lost our familiar shortcomings. The experience of doing our inventory showed us that our negativity and fears were unfounded. We discovered that being honest with ourselves was better than living a lie.

If we experienced discomfort while preparing our Fourth Step inventory, or if we were triggered by strong emotions or lust, we picked up the phone and sought support and direction from our sponsor or other recovering members. We reviewed or reworked Step Two and remembered that God would not abandon us. We reviewed Step Three where we had decided, among other things, that letting God lead us through the Steps would be better than continuing to run our life our way. We prayed and tried again. Some of us found it helpful to do this work in the presence of other members, or to do it in small, daily chunks rather than attempting an hours-long marathon of inventory writing. We were encouraged and reminded that this venture was a process of self-discovery that promised us a new life of humility, faith, and fulfillment.

While some believe that a lot of sobriety is necessary before tackling Step Four, we follow the guidance in the book *Alcoholics Anonymous*, which recommends doing Step Four "at once" after taking Step Three. Bill W., co-founder of Alcoholics Anonymous, did a Fourth Step inventory just a few days after his last drink, while still in the hospital. It is possible to find many reasons to procrastinate on this work, but we found that delay thwarted our spiritual growth and created an opportunity for relapse.

Writing a Fourth Step Inventory does not need to be a lengthy drawn-out process, but many of us are daunted by the prospect. Therefore, we benefited from regularly scheduled periods of writing our inventory—daily if possible. Five or ten minutes each day was far better than longer periods once or twice a month. We needed to practice recovery every day, and this was the best way to move through Step Four. Thus, we were encouraged by our progress.

While our work had to be thorough, we avoided perfectionism, as it would delay completion, perhaps indefinitely. No Fourth Step inventory would be perfect or include everything. We did our best and trusted that God, working through our sponsor or another person, would provide us what we needed. "Let go and let God" applies particularly to this Step.

The value of doing a written Fourth Step inventory cannot be overstated. We put down on paper in our own words an honest and thorough appraisal of our behavior, character defects, and assets. Complete sentences, good grammar, and good penmanship were not necessary. This act of writing paid big dividends. We began to see what was really going on inside us. We were uncovering our strengths and weaknesses, directly and honestly. We were gaining insight that we never had before.

Step Four was the beginning of a lifelong process of self-appraisal and accountability. As we continued on this path, we would have many more opportunities to review our conduct, motives, shortcomings, and strengths. The Fourth Step inventory and Fifth Step sharing gave us tools to use any time we were emotionally disturbed and assailed by resentment, fear, shame, guilt, remorse, self-loathing, self-pity, or pride. This Step marked the path of meaningful and ongoing recovery.

"Clear away the wreckage of your past," *Alcoholics Anonymous* tells us (164). Step Four helped us begin that task. Here we identified the wreckage that had been dragging us down for years. We learned how we had been assigning blame indiscriminately to ourselves and others. We saw both our character flaws and our assets with a more realistic perspective. We grew in self-acceptance. We began to develop a level of honesty that we had only hoped for or glimpsed. We were learning what must change if our relations with others were to improve. We looked forward to being free of our burdens by giving them away in Step Five.

## *Members of SA Share*

### *1*

Taking other peoples' inventories rather than my own was my favorite pastime. I was soul-sick and knew deep inside the terrible things I had done. So I had to go through life with a magnifying glass focused on others. I couldn't stand to look at myself honestly. Denial of my harmful behavior drove me to immerse myself in fantasy rather than reality. So I didn't examine myself. I needed to live in the illusion that I was the victim.

Little did I know that the cure for my illness was a mirror, not a magnifying glass. It was vital for me to see the wrongs I did to others. I was a prisoner of the illusion that my behavior toward others was justified by how others treated me. Only a new level of honesty could free me. This was a crucial change in my attitude.

This change came about, not through a lot of thought and insight, but through writing out my Fourth Step inventory. I was guided by my Higher Power and a sponsor who had worked the Steps.

*2*

Shame was my biggest block to working Step Four. I believed I was all bad, with no redeeming qualities whatsoever. I told myself that the inventory I was writing proved I was no good so I might as well act out. I would not stay sober. Lust didn't want me to find my strengths.

My sponsor helped me initially by telling me that his Higher Power only made wonderful human beings. I needed to hear that. He said people might be able to hide their finer points but that, sooner or later, if they made a Third Step decision and worked the other Steps, these would begin to show through. He said that it was important for me to balance my inventory with some of my assets no matter how hard they were for me to find. He helped me see that I had the courage to try, the willingness to ask for help. I had the desire to survive, to be part of the group, and to be helpful to others. I had intelligence, a sense of humor, education, faith, and a conscience.

With his encouragement and God's power, I was able to stay sober. I completed my inventory and identified many areas I was willing to change and get help with. At the same time, I was able to capitalize on some of my strengths to help me get through the process. Sometimes I still struggle with self-loathing, but Step Four has given me tools to keep me from being overwhelmed by it.

*3*

My sponsor told me I was ready to start my Fourth Step inventory. He told me how powerful this Step could be. The first question I addressed was, "Where had I failed to take responsibility?" I thought it would be a fairly short list. When the pages continued to fill, it became apparent how my actions and character defects had damaged my life and the lives of those around me. I was appalled and frightened. Lust magnified my flaws and prevented me from seeing any of my positive qualities. I was unable to find any balance. I wanted to act out. I reached for the phone instead.

My sponsor reassured me that my response was not unusual. He suggested that I take things slowly and be close to a phone when writing. However, the fear generated by my near slip led me to conclude that I should stop writing!

As the weeks slipped by, my sponsor repeatedly asked me when I would be finished with my inventory. I would respond, "It's coming along." One night, my sponsor confronted me. If I wasn't willing to work the Steps, he didn't need to be my sponsor. I was resentful of being called on my arrogance, but I knew he was right.

I came to understand that if I wanted recovery, I could not do it alone. I needed to follow my sponsor's direction. I had to go back to Step Three, to surrender my will, fear, and procrastination to my Higher Power. Once I did this I was able to regain my focus and complete my Fourth Step inventory.

*4*

I was the one the book *Alcoholics Anonymous* described as having such great knowledge of all the inner workings of his own mind. I had been the one in the meeting room who could share so eloquently about all of the psychological stuff he had read. With absolutely no advance notice, my self-powered program of recovery ran out of gas, and I found myself immersed in the world of internet pornography. After twenty months of sobriety, I accepted a twenty-four hour chip. For the first time since joining SA, I didn't have the right thing to say.

I knew something was wrong but couldn't figure out what it was. Figuring things out was how I functioned. What I didn't know was that in working my own plan, I was simply creating a whole new version of the same old me. I was attempting to use a sick mind to fix a sick mind.

The key to my freedom was revealed on page 67 of *Alcoholics Anonymous*: "Referring to our list again. Putting out of our minds the wrongs others had done, we resolutely looked for our own mistakes." Disregarding others' behaviors entirely, I looked for where my actions had been selfish, dishonest, self-seeking, and frightened, and put these on paper. This process added an essential dimension to this Step which had been missing. I couldn't get sober until I stopped using my knowledge as my Higher Power.

*5*

Completing a fear inventory in Step Four (*AA* 68) ushered in a significant awakening in my life. I realized that even though I didn't know it, I had been living in fear, and most of my actions were based on that.

I learned that my fear is usually worse than the object of my fear. In a few cases, when I surrendered it to my Higher Power, the thing I feared came to pass. Yet, it was never as bad as I had expected. The fear-based insanity that I put myself through was much worse.

I also learned that I give power to something by fearing it. For some weird reason, when I get caught up in fear and let it direct my actions, my actions tend to increase the likelihood of the feared event. In many cases, after I surrender to my Higher Power, the thing I fear loses power and does not occur.

*6*

I have done repeated Fourth Step inventories. Each time, I have discovered subtle nuances in my emotional make up that I had not noticed in previous inventories. For me, working the Steps is more of a process than an event. As I discover these more subtle character defects, I write about them, then give them away to the God of my understanding and to my sponsor. This is the way I begin to free myself of the power they have over me.

*7*

I came into SA weighed down by constantly carrying two large sacks of rocks everywhere I went. One sack represents all of my resentments about things that happened to me in the past. The other sack represents all of my fears about the things that might happen to me in the future. Step Four helps me identify each rock, so that in later Steps I can lay every one of them down and leave them behind. The Program teaches me how to stop picking up new rocks. Oh my God! That's what peace and serenity feels like? I never knew.

*8*

There is a pot of gold inside me. It is always glowing, but it is covered with garbage. As the garbage is removed one piece at a time, more of the glow can show through. Steps Four and Five help identify the garbage. Steps Six and Seven remove the garbage. It is just that simple.

For years I did not understand this principle. My sponsor would often say to me, "Maybe someday your intelligence will catch up to your education." The problem is that my addict shares my brain with me. It has the same intelligence, but it always lies. If I listen to my addict, it will always win. I am learning not to listen to the lies, but instead to listen to that intuitive inner voice.

*9*

I began to believe that I could walk through the jungle of my twisted life and come out free—only because I saw others do it before me. Step meetings, the affirmations of the God of my understanding, the reassurance of my sponsor, and hearing others' stories of relief and even joy after giving their Fifth Step gave me courage. I had been stuck on writing my Fourth Step inventory. Somehow a miracle happened, a change of attitude. I just began writing. Nothing seemed to help change my life until I wrote it all down and gave it away to another human being and to a God I had finally come to trust. Through the acceptance of those in the program, I experienced the forgiveness and love of my Higher Power. Completion of Steps Four and Five brought relief, balance, and a sense of self that included calm, acceptance, fellowship, and humor. I couldn't see where I had been until I was somewhere else!

*10*

I was beginning to make progress in turning over my resentments. Most were pet peeves with which I had chosen to take issue. I learned I could just choose to not let these issues bother me.

My difficulty was those deep-seated resentments which I came to call justified resentments. These always began with others doing something to me. Their actions caused me pain and as a result I felt justified in those resentments. I believed that they needed to make an amends to me!

Because they had hurt me, I had concluded that I was a victim of their actions. I therefore was not responsible. I was justified, and they needed to correct the problem. My only recourse was to isolate from them in order to protect myself from any additional pain they might cause me by their actions.

I subsequently learned that "whenever I am disturbed, no matter what the cause, there is something wrong" *with me.* Thus I needed to identify my role in every interaction with my fellows that caused me pain. As I dug deeper with the help of my sponsor, I began to understand that the actions of some had struck at my ego or fears, causing me pain. My immediate reaction to this pain was to be a victim and blame them for the pain I was feeling.

In recovery, my role is to deflate my ego or confront my fears. I needed to identify the cause of the pain that was disturbing me and own my side of the problem. Once I became aware of my defects at work, and only then, could I be in a position to accept the situation and surrender it to my Higher Power.

*11*

When I worked Step Four, my sponsor had very clear directions. "Don't psychoanalyze yourself! You are simply making lists. We will figure out together what it all means when you share everything with me in Step Five." I found that to be very valuable advice. Today, I share the same caution with my sponsees. We are not searching for reasons, excuses, blame, shame, or underlying psychological causes. We are learning to take a thorough, honest inventory—to see ourselves as we really are, knowing that we don't have to stay that way any longer.

## *Step into Action*

### *Recommended Readings*

We suggest that members read and study the following before working the Step:

*Alcoholics Anonymous* (*AA*)
"Chapter 5" 63 - 71

*Sexaholics Anonymous* (*SA*)
"Making the Wrongs Right" 97 - 104
*"Step Four"* 105 - 110

*Twelve Steps and Twelve Traditions* (*12&12*)
"Step Four" 42

## *One Method of Working Step Four And Some Questions to Consider*

There are many good ways to do a Fourth Step inventory. The method described below is largely based on the recommendations in *Alcoholics Anonymous* (63-70).

We look at our resentments, our fears, and the harms we did to others, including our sexual misconduct. Whenever we prepare to write, we find it helpful to pray the Third Step prayer and ask for God's guidance. As we write, we keep in contact with our sponsor, letting him or her review our writing at regular intervals. Indeed, this writing may require several sessions.

### *Resentment Toward People, Institutions, and Principles*

In a spiral notebook, we make a list of all the people with whom we are angry or resentful. Some of us do this chronologically from birth, and some begin with the people in our immediate lives. When we have prayed and sat with no new names coming up, we turn to a new page and write a list of institutions at which we are angry. Some examples of institutions are banks, schools, marriage, or the government. Other examples include groups of people (rich people, poor people) and ideologies (religions and philosophies of life). We repeat the process for principles we resent. Principles include abstractions like authority, life, or death; activities, like doing housework or balancing a checkbook; and proverbial truths, like "Waste not, want not" or "Handsome is as handsome does."

When the lists are finished, we look at the chart on page 65 of *Alcoholics Anonymous.* We open a spiral notebook to two blank facing pages. At the left side of the left hand page, we write the heading, "I'm resentful at." We title a second column on the left page, "The cause."

In column one, we write the name of the first person on the list. Next to that name, in column two, we write our resentment, for example, "He shamed me in front of others" or "She has a husband and children." If referring to a complex incident (for example, from childhood) we write a brief descriptive note. A few words are plenty for us and our Higher Power to know what we are talking about. We are brief and specific; fifteen words per resentment is a good guideline. If we need to journal to become clear about why we're angry, we can do that in another place and bring a brief summary back to this column. We go through each entry on the list and write whatever resentments come up for each one. We work from top to bottom so that columns one and two are complete before moving on to column three, which we label "Affects my."

In most cases we find that we are angry because some part of our self is threatened. In column three we list what instinct this person, institution, or principle threatens. Usually self-esteem, emotional security, personal relationships, sexual relationships, financial security, pride, and ambition are where we feel at risk. Sometimes we are aware that we have fear, apprehension, anxiety, uneasiness, or dread related to a particular resentment. If so, we also include "fear" in column three.

| *I'm resentful at:* | *The cause:* | *Affects my:* |
|---|---|---|
| my boss | he put me down in front of the others | self-esteem<br>security ambitions<br>personal relations(fear) |
| | he yells when I come in late | Pride<br>self-esteem<br>security<br>ambitions<br>personal relations<br>pride<br>(fear) |

| *I'm resentful at:* | *The cause:* | *Affects my:* |
|---|---|---|
| the Main St. Bank | wouldn't let me open an account | security (fear)<br>self-esteem<br>ambition<br>personal relations |

| | | |
|---|---|---|
| medical system | poor treatment result | self-esteem<br>security<br>personal relations<br>(fear) |
| good-looking people | have it easy, can date whomever they want | self-esteem<br>security<br>personal relations<br>ambition<br>sex relations<br>(fear) |
| life on life's terms | it's too hard | self-esteem<br>security<br>ambition<br>(fear) |

In *Alcoholics Anonymous* (66) we learn that we are unable to get rid of our resentments on our own, and that our lives are at risk from them if we don't. The solution is prayer coupled with action. This prayer takes a variety of forms, but usually reminds us that those we resent, like ourselves, are learning by making mistakes. By surrendering these resentments to our Higher Power through prayer while we write our inventory, we are gradually relieved of our resentments. As we work on our Fourth Step inventory, we pray for those on our list, even if we don't want to. By repeatedly turning over our resentments to our Higher Power, eventually we find that we can sincerely wish well for each person, institution, and principle on our list.

The bottom of page 66 says, "We realized that the people who wronged us were perhaps spiritually sick." An AA oldtimer defined "spiritually sick" as "cut off from God."

Think of the 3 worst things you have done in your life. Had you been walking in the "sunlight of the spirit," in close contact with God, could you have done those things? You probably wouldn't even have thought of them in His Presence. This observation can help you see that those who wronged you were sick too.

With your own ugliest mistakes in mind, take as much time as you need to pray for each individual on your list as follows:

"God, please help me to see that George was just spiritually sick when he did those things to me."

"God, please help me to see that Mary was just spiritually sick when she did those things to me."

Continue in this fashion until you've prayed the list once, no matter what your results are.

The following excerpt from *Alcoholics Anonymous* describes a method an oldtimer found to resolve a longstanding resentment that was not completely resolved by her Step work:

> If you have a resentment you want to be free of, if you will pray for the person or the thing that you resent, you will be free. If you will ask in prayer for everything you want for yourself to be given to them, you will be free. Ask for their health, their prosperity, their happiness, and you will be free. Even when you don't really want it for them and your prayers are only words and you don't mean it, go ahead and do it anyway. Do it every day for two weeks, and you will find you have come to mean it and to want it for them, and you will realize that where you used to feel bitterness and resentment and hatred, you now feel compassionate understanding and love (*AA* 552).

The experience of many members is that two weeks may not be enough time. Don't worry about how long it takes. Just keep praying.

Pray this prayer anytime you think any of the things that angered you, and set aside specific times each week to devote to this prayer.

Once we have written out the causes and "affects" for all the people on our list, we do the same for the institutions and principles.

Remember that we don't have to mean it. We have only been asked to pray it. We may even choose to begin our prayers with something like: "God, I probably won't mean a word of this, but I really need to be free of this old hate I am harboring against some of your other children. So here goes." As we finish praying for each individual, we ask, "Do I really mean it?" If we keep working on this exercise, eventually the answer will be "yes."

Resentment is like ice around my heart. By praying, I can hold the icy heart up to the Sunlight of the Spirit. The ice has a thickness based on the severity of the events and how much I have fed the resentment. But no matter how thick, Sunlight will eventually melt ice.

My sponsor said that what I really wanted was mercy for myself and justice for everyone else. But our only real options are mercy for everyone OR justice for everyone. I am part of everyone, and I get to choose. I know that I need mercy rather than justice, so I have chosen mercy for everyone.

When our first three columns and prayer work are complete, we are ready to look for our mistakes. We use the right hand page of our notebook and label it "My mistake." If it is not clear to us where we are wrong, we describe where we have been selfish (what did we want and why?); dishonest (what lies did we tell ourselves or others? what is the real truth?); self-seeking (what did we do to get what we wanted? how did we react?); and frightened (what were we afraid of?). These questions will point to our wrongdoing in most circumstances. Using the example of the resentment against the boss, we wrote about our mistake on the right-hand page.

My mistake (on right hand page):

*Selfish*—what did I want and why?

I wanted him to be kind so I could feel good about myself and be liked by the others.

*Dishonest*—what was the real truth?

I couldn't control him or the situation; I took it personally even though he did this to everyone; I've done the same thing to others; I didn't try very hard on my last assignment; it was not his job to make me feel good about myself; his actions were irrelevant to being liked by the others.

*Self-seeking*—what did I do to get what I wanted? how did I react?
blame, criticize, judge, bristle, sulk, withdraw, gossip, take a long lunch, rant and rave, sneer, roll my eyes, people-please him, grit my teeth, do damage control with other staff, beat up on myself

*Frightened*—what was I afraid of?
others' opinions, being embarrassed, not being respected

## *Fear*

Next we make a list of our fears on a new page. Fear can mean worry, anxiety, or full-blown panic. This list can include almost anything: people, principles, institutions, fantasies, powers greater than ourselves. We list fears from our resentment inventory (columns three or four) as well as others.

We turn the page, and for each fear we answer the following questions in a few sentences:

1. Why did I have this fear? What was I afraid of? Am I threatened? Was I overly sensitive from something long past?

2. How has self-reliance failed me? How have I tried to manage this fear, and how has that made things worse? Have my actions and my attempts to run the show myself reinforced and fed my fear?

3. How could trusting and relying upon God help me deal with this fear?

After we have answered these questions we refer back to *Alcoholics Anonymous*: "We ask Him to remove our fear and direct our attention to what He would have us be. At once, we commence to outgrow fear." (*AA* 68).

We find that, once again, prayer coupled with action is the solution. We use prayer to address each fear. We begin to see ourselves as people who can live in faith, not fear; who can start the day with hope, not despair; who can take the next right action, rather than wallow in the expectation of defeat. This is how we begin to outgrow fear.

For each fear we write our current understanding of what God would have us be. We need a change of attitude, not more self-willed efforts to fix the problem. We often find that we already have these qualities, although they may be overshadowed by our shortcomings. We continue to pray for further understanding of what God would have us be, and we pray for help to be that. An example follows:

| | |
|---|---|
| *Fear:* | The husband of a woman with whom I had an affair will hurt me. |
| *Why do I have it?* | He is a violent alcoholic who owns firearms, and has threatened to get revenge. |
| *How has self-reliance failed me?* | I feel paranoid. I make complex plans about how to avoid him. I have caller ID so I don't answer his calls. I feel doomed because if he wants to find me, he can. I can't protect my family. |
| *How could trusting and relying upon God help?* | I realize that I cannot control it. I trust that whatever happens will be arranged by God so that it is the best thing that could happen for everyone involved and is just what each of us needs. |
| *What would God have me be?* | Honest and humble. Kind, considerate, and respectful of the husband and others. Trusting that if we meet it will be for good purpose, and I will be well prepared. |

Some of us find that we have fears that recur. One technique we use is to write these fears on an index card and number them. For example:

1. I will fail in my job.
2. Financial insecurity—I will lose all.
3. I am an inadequate wife and mother.

On the flip side of the card we write what we believe God would have us be. For each of the numbered fears we have a numbered response:

1. Honest, industrious, considerate
2. Frugal, industrious, trusting in Him to provide
3. Self-caring, loving, considerate

We keep this card with us so that when we are assailed by fear, we can refer to the card and ask for our Higher Power's help. For example, when I am afraid of losing my job, I am reminded to pray: "Please relieve me of this fear of losing my job, and help me be an honest, industrious employee, considerate of my coworkers."

### *Sexual Conduct and Personal Relations*

> Now about sex. . . .
> We reviewed our own conduct over the years past. Where had we been selfish, dishonest, or inconsiderate? Whom had we hurt? Did we unjustifiably arouse jealousy, suspicion or bitterness? Where were we at fault, what should we have done instead? We got this all down on paper and looked at it (*AA* 68 -9).

We make a list of people with whom we have had sexual or romantic relations. Since we wrote a First Step Inventory as one of the first writing exercises in beginning to work the Steps, we already have a list to draw from. For each situation we answer the above questions in a few sentences. Here is an example:

| | |
|---|---|
| *Who:* | Person I had an affair with |
| *Where was I selfish?* | I was sexually demanding and promiscuous. I was not committed to the relationship even though the other person was emotionally involved. |
| *Where was I dishonest?* | I lied about my feelings to get what I wanted. I used emotional involvement to manipulate. |
| *Where was I inconsiderate?* | Our relationship resulted in the breakup of my partner's marriage, causing much pain for spouse and children. |
| *Whom did I hurt?* | My partner, parents, friend. |
| *Where did I arouse jealousy?* | I flirted openly and talked about other partners. |
| *Where did I arouse suspicion?* | I was unreliable and made excuses for my absences. |
| *Where did I arouse bitterness?* | I raged and blamed my partner for our problems. |
| *Where was I at fault?* | I didn't treat my partner with respect. I used my partner for sex. I was emotionally and verbally abusive. |
| *What should I have done instead?* | I should have treated my partner as a friend. I should not have had sex with my partner. I should have allowed an emotional and spiritual relationship to develop. I should have sought sexual sobriety. |

Those of us who have acted out anonymously find it useful to write about prostitutes or anonymous partners collectively in a single paragraph. We use the questions to identify recurring themes. If there were painful, disgusting, or arousing episodes that trigger us, we address them with our sponsor. We make our list as thorough as possible. Keeping secrets might lead us to a relapse.

> In this way we tried to shape a sane and sound ideal for our future sex life. … We asked God to mold our ideals and help us live up to them. (*AA* 69).

We review this work, especially our answers to the last question, "What should we have done instead?" After prayer and reflection, we write about our ideal in regard to our future sexual conduct and review this with our sponsor. We can write this in the form of a list, a prayer, or a letter to God. An example follows:

- I surrender my sex life to my Higher Power.
- I will not have a sexual or romantic relationship with anyone other than my spouse.
- I will only engage in physical sexual intimacy when it is based on emotional and spiritual intimacy.
- I will avoid physical sexual intimacy when I am lusting, angry, afraid, or otherwise triggered and will not use it as a form of manipulation.
- I will not use lust as a drug.

We find that we can apply these questions to all of our relationships even where there was no romantic or sexual involvement. In this way, we are able to get a clear picture of all the people we have harmed.

If there are other situations that bother us but don't appear to fit under one of our three inventories—resentment, fear, and sexual conduct and personal relations—we make note of them and discuss them with our sponsor. When we have completed these written inventories, we are ready for Step Five.

# *Step Five*

## *Admitted to God, to ourselves, and to another human being the exact nature of our wrongs*

The Fifth Step is the act of giving away our Fourth Step inventory. To gain maximum benefit from writing our First Step inventory––a history of the thinking and behavior that brought us to SA—we shared it with our group. In a similar way, gaining maximum benefit from writing a searching and fearless moral inventory required that we share it with another human being. For us, Step Five thus became a giant step on the road to integrity. We were beginning to practice being the same person on the outside as we were on the inside. Working the first four Steps had given us a new perspective on our lives. In Step Five, as we opened ourselves to another person, we left our lives of spiritual isolation behind.

Our Fourth Step inventory showed us exactly where we had been wrong and how we had caused problems in our relations with others. It also showed where our shortcomings had overshadowed our assets. In Step Five we faced our weaknesses, difficulties, and strengths and shared them with God and with another human being. This opened the door to an entirely different way of living where we no longer needed to hide. We found that leading with our weakness and being open and honest about our shortcomings created intimacy in our lives and made us more useful to others. Living life from a foundation of honesty and transparency was easier and felt better than hiding.

If we were apprehensive at the prospect of discussing our shortcomings with another person, we were reminded of our willingness to go to any lengths for a spiritual experience. We found it was necessary to share all of ourselves for several reasons:

- Another person, familiar with our story and condition, was able to see our work from a different perspective. Perhaps we were not being honest with ourselves. That person could see our mistakes, exaggerations, irrational thinking, and strengths where we could not.

- Sharing our wrongs with another has long been a powerful method of ego deflation. As our condition is one of self-centeredness, this was necessary for our renewed health and spiritual growth.

- As we shared these secrets with another, they began to lose their power. We learned at some deep level that we didn't need to hide from God, from ourselves, or from other people. The shame, fear, and anger that drove us to lust began to leave.

- Perhaps the most important reason was that we might relapse if we were not completely honest about ourselves with someone else; thus, we risked our recovery, our marriages and children, our chances for more meaningful relationships and pursuits, and ultimately our lives (*AA* 72-3).

We had felt separated from others by a "mysterious barrier we could neither surmount nor understand" (*12 & 12* 57). We didn't feel that we fit into society, community, or family. We didn't feel that our needs were met or that our accomplishments were adequately appreciated. We isolated ourselves further in lives of fantasy and acting out, detached and distracted by our lust. Entering the Fellowship, we were relieved to find others like us, but we still felt separated from the world. We feared abandonment and rejection if another human being really knew our hidden inner self. As we gave away our Fifth Step and experienced acceptance from another person who heard our darkest secrets, we began to realize we were not alone. Our defects and motives were not unique. As we accepted ourselves as we really were, we began to break down our lifelong pattern of isolation. We were able to be present for ourselves and others.

Seeing our lives through the eyes of another, without judgment or fear, helped us see what sort of influence we had on the people and events of our past. This was the beginning of integrity and humility. Both exaggeration and denial of our mistakes began to fade. We no longer needed to swing between grandiosity and despair. We saw that we were actually imperfect and worthwhile members of the human race. We began to be more honest about ourselves and to take up residence in reality. Released from the mental posturing of the past, we could grow into the person our Higher Power would have us be.

Before working the Steps, we had made a fine art of keeping score, but now we were feeling compassion and even forgiveness. We began to consider the possibility that we could be forgiven. If we could find forgiveness toward others, perhaps we could be granted acceptance and forgiveness of ourselves.

Most of us never really believed that our sponsors had been as sick as we were. But as they shared similar experiences, as we did with them, we glimpsed the progress they had made. We imagined that the recovery they found was possible for us too. Hope brightened and our faith grew. We believed that a Power greater than ourselves could actually change us and teach us to live and behave differently. We saw that God's plan for our lives had to be better than the best we could do.

Miracles do happen in recovery, and Step Five is one of them. This Step changed us, perhaps not all at once or with a flash of lightning, but we could feel the difference between the old life and the new. Our feelings of separateness and isolation diminished. We sensed a Power greater than ourselves acting in our lives. When we surrendered our secrets, when we came out of hiding, we opened ourselves to God's grace and to communion with the human race.

## *Members of SA Share*

### *1*

There are three admissions in Step Five—one to myself, one to God, and one to another human being. The admission to myself is for honesty, a way to break through my own veil of denial. The admission to God is for forgiveness. The admission to another human being is for humility. Honesty, forgiveness, and humility are three traits I did not bring with me to SA. They are traits that I needed to learn.

In my own experience, by the time I admit to myself and to God the exact nature of my wrongs, I am more than ready to admit them to another human being. I have always chosen my sponsor to be my "other human being," but that has been my choice. Some people I have sponsored have chosen to go to others to make this admission. I believe there is only one wrong way to do this Step, and that is to not do it at all.

*2*

I began my first Fourth Step at a difficult time in my life when I was almost one year sober. At the time there were no other women in my group with sobriety or experience whom I could turn to for help. What I did was make a list of all of my defects of character with short notes describing each. My list of defects and related notes ran to several pages. It was compiled over several sessions of reflection while alone in a quiet place.

For Step Five, I used these short notes to share with my sponsor at much greater length and depth. Her insights were helpful. She helped me see that related to each of my character defects were complementary potential character assets. I felt tremendous relief and freedom. I had a new awareness of a Power greater than myself helping me to grow and change.

Now, years later, I have done several Fifth Steps using different methods. I always strive for completeness, but as the fog clears, I always see more things that should have been included but weren't. This narrowing of the path is a wonderful thing to look forward to.

*3*

Step Five required courage. I had to bring into the light the thoughts and deeds I wanted to keep hidden. When I lived in lust, I hid my worst behavior from others for fear of what they would think. I hid the extent of my obsession even from myself by a kind of selective amnesia, and I reinterpreted my behavior to make it seem more acceptable. I kept God out of the picture. I was invested in a great cover-up. Through years of obsessive thinking and behavior, I built a wall to hide my secrets, to keep control, to keep others out. That was the life of isolation that Step Five invited me to leave behind.

Completion of Step Four required a lot of writing and prayer. Through this work I gained a different perspective on many of the events and people in my life. Some of my resentments and fears evaporated upon writing them down, while others seemed to intensify. In some instances, I was unable to find my mistake, while in others I exaggerated my responsibility. Sometimes I was relieved that my resentments, fears, and harms were finite in number, and other times I was amazed that there were so many.

Once I had finished my Fourth Step inventory, I began worrying about how my sponsor would react to some of the things I had done, especially the sexual harms. I was afraid he would be disgusted and refuse to work with me anymore. As we went through the inventory, he showed me how selfishness, fear, and dishonesty had led to those actions I found so shameful. He asked me if I was willing to grow out of these defects and live my life by a new set of principles. Indeed, I was. He reminded me that God had been with me throughout my life and loved me enough to bring me to SA. He asked if I was ready to accept God's forgiveness and direction. When I said yes, I felt as though I had joined the human race. I was no longer alone!

*4*

I presented my written Fourth Step inventory to my sponsor, and we reviewed it together. She saw patterns that had eluded me. She pointed out where I overlooked selfishness, dishonesty, self-seeking, or fear. She guided me to see motives that I hid from myself. She saw where I demonstrated love, courage, or other admirable traits. She reminded me that these inventories identified my assets as well as my liabilities.

I try to provide similarly useful feedback to my sponsees. While I am willing to confront denial, dishonesty, or manipulative behavior, I also want to affirm willingness, honesty, and courage. I believe that even in the depths of our disease, each of us tried to choose the least destructive options we saw at the time. As we learn better options, we improve. I need to let go of my shame for not knowing what I had never been taught or shown, and I need to support others as they learn to do the same. I frequently share an example of my own poor choices to let my sponsee know she is not unique. When my sponsee is finished, I generally ask if there is anything else that she has been too afraid or too ashamed to share. I remind her that we are as sick as our secrets. Once she has shared her Fourth Step inventory with me, withholding nothing, we review the Step Five promises (*AA* 75).

*5*

When I did Step Five for the first time, I went over to my sponsor's house and read my Fourth Step inventory to him. It was a very beneficial exercise for me. Reading aloud all the resentments, fears, and harms showed me clearly the patterns that had been forged in my behaviors and attitudes. Even though I was intimately familiar with what I had written, I was horrified to hear myself recite behaviors and attitudes of a very different person from the one I had hoped to become.

My sponsor fell asleep several times during my reading, and I had to make loud noises to wake him up. I was annoyed by this at first, but I soon realized how good it was for me to have to exert myself (with a loud voice and occasional noises) to give my resentments, fears, and harms away to him. He commented from time to time, and when I was finished we had a good talk about the whole thing: all the ploys, pretenses, and dishonesty I had practiced to deal with people and with life.

I felt elated when we had finished, as if a great weight had been lifted off of me. I felt as if I had really done some good work for myself. I was grateful for my sponsor, his insights, and his genuine concern for me.

*6*

When I finally set up a time to do Step Five with my sponsor, I began to worry that I had not done a good enough job. When I shared this with my sponsor, she asked if I had listed perfectionism as part of my inventory. We laughed together at the obviousness of my defect. I was able to proceed without the critical voice in my head that was my usual companion.

As I shared the nature of my wrongs, my sponsor would challenge me to elaborate on what the positive side of each trait might look like. At first, I could see no redeeming features. With her help, I began to understand how my stubbornness could at times be perseverance; that my perfectionism helped me perform quality work on my job. Each examination gave me a fuller picture of what was truly stocked on my shelves. Contrary to my initial assessment, my inventory was not all damaged goods. As I continue to grow in this program, I am reminded to take inventory regularly to make sure that my view of my stock is accurate.

*7*

Over the years of trudging this Road of Happy Destiny, I have learned that I have to continue practicing the principle of Step Five every day. It is not just a one-time sharing of my Fourth Step with my sponsor. I call this principle "Telling on myself." For a sexaholic like me, secrets can kill. I have found that if I tell on myself to my sponsor, to a recovery friend, or in a meeting—if I share what is happening in my life or what is going on in my head, then those things lose their power over me. Any time I think "They don't need to know that," I risk my serenity and recovery.

In Step Four I learned the principle of self-inventory—how to see the truth about myself. But if I keep that truth to myself, or even just between me and God, I can still deceive myself. Step Five teaches me the importance of sharing with another sexaholic. If I don't tell on myself, then victory over my next lust temptation depends completely on my state of surrender and connection to God. If I honestly share my struggles with my recovery friends, it not only strengthens my spiritual condition, it reminds me that I'm not in this alone. I have a band of brothers and sisters who have my back.

*8*

I learned the ability to admit my wrongs by going to meetings. When somebody in a meeting voices the despair he or she feels about our addiction and goes underneath to voice the causes of the despair, I learned to have the courage to do the same. The guidance of my sponsor, however, was critical to recognizing my wrongs. Previously, I had thought that a complete moral inventory was a list of all the wrongs I had committed. My sponsor gently reminded me that it is not a list of wrongs. It is a list of resentments and fears. Only by digging into my emotions was I able to go deeper and uncover the underlying wrong, the character defect that produced the wrong behaviors I was becoming more easily able to admit. This emotional inventory taking, now done daily as part of my Tenth Step, is perhaps the most significant recovery skill I've learned from my sponsor.

*9*

I put off finishing my Fourth Step because I was afraid to share it with my sponsor in Step Five. I dreaded going through my list of resentments, fears, and wrongs with someone else. When the day finally came, I was surprised to find out how freeing this Step really was. Within five minutes I began to experience the freedom that accompanies getting thoroughly honest with someone else. As I shared my defects I quickly saw that, "surrendering them broke the power they had over [me]" (*SA* 205). As I finished, I was awed by the sense of peace I felt. For the first time since early childhood, I felt connected to another human being and my creator.

*10*

Giving Step Four away was a real breakthrough in this program for me. It helped reveal what was behind my acting out behaviors. There were emotional issues for which acting out provided an immediate escape. Step Four helped me become more emotionally attuned. Working with my sponsor, I identified patterns that we later worked on in more depth as part of Steps Six and Seven. My sponsor demonstrated kindness and sympathy and identified with many of my issues. He also pointed out a couple of areas he thought I should give more serious examination—things I did not see very well on my own.

Through this acceptance and release of the wreckage of my past, I experienced the presence of God entering my life. My sponsor indicated it was helpful to him to be of service.

*11*

Giving away my Fifth Step was a life-changing spiritual experience for me. When my sponsor fell asleep while I was sharing it, I didn't get resentful. I believe I was giving away my resentments. No, I took it as a sign from my Higher Power that:

1. He had heard it all before;
2. He already knew all my stuff (I was the one who needed to learn about me)—and
3. My Higher Power accepts me for who I am and still loves me.

God is surely *for* the sexaholic!

*12*

From other members of SA, I learned that some sponsors, when listening to a sponsee share their inventories, pray for each person or institution the sponsee had harmed in some way.

So, when a sponsee gives away their Step Four inventory to me, the Step Five experience has become a very spiritual event for me. Our prayers for the people they have harmed humanizes those people and prepares the sponsee for Steps Eight, Nine, and Ten. This is our basic prayer… "Higher Power, bless ______. Meet their needs. May your will be done in their life."

## *Step into Action*

### *Recommended Readings*

We suggest that members read and study the following before working the Step:

*Alcoholics Anonymous* (*AA*)
"Chapter 6" 72-75

*Sexaholics Anonymous* (*SA*)
"Step Five" 111-114

*Twelve Steps and Twelve Traditions* (*12&12*)
"Step Five" 55-62

## *One Method of Working Step Five*

We choose a safe person to hear our Fifth Step according to the guidelines in the Recommended Readings. Usually it is our sponsor.

Some of us are directed to share our inventory first with our Higher Power, in prayer, at a place we consider sacred. This might be a house of worship, meeting place, meditation room, or outside in nature where we feel we could meet the God of our understanding. Next we take time to review the inventory again with ourselves. Finally, we schedule a lengthy, open-ended time to meet and share with our sponsor or other person we have chosen. Others of us share our inventory only once, with another person. We may have another chair or a candle present to remind us that we are also sharing with our Higher Power.

This is a very special time. Whenever possible, we suggest starting early in the day to allow ample time for discussion. Many have taken the Step at the home of the sponsor or sponsee. Fifth Steps have also been successfully taken in places of worship, parks, or other places where there is privacy. Restaurants and other public places are usually not suitable for Step Five. Fifth Steps are done by phone when long distances prevent us from meeting face-to-face.

These sessions are often opened with prayer and readings from recovery or other spiritual literature (for example, *AA* 72-75). We share our inventory, our histories, and ourselves completely. We keep no secrets. It is necessary to be thorough if we want to live useful, meaningful lives and grow.

As sponsors hearing another's Fourth Step inventory, we share insights, perspective and, where relevant, our own experience. We keep the discussion moving and focused on Step Five. We find that, by helping others, we often have new insights about our own character. We try to be honest and supportive, expressing acceptance, encouragement, and gratitude.

When finished, we share a prayer of thanks and review the Fifth Step promises:

> Once we have taken this step, withholding nothing, we are delighted. We can look the world in the eye. We can be alone at perfect peace and ease. Our fears fall from us. We begin to feel the nearness of our Creator. We may have had certain spiritual beliefs, but now we begin to have a spiritual experience. The feeling that the [lust] problem has disappeared will often come strongly. We feel we are on the Broad Highway, walking hand in hand with the Spirit of the Universe (*AA* 75).

Then we proceed with the second portion of Step Five. This is a process of review and reflection which is described in the last paragraph on page 75 in *Alcoholics Anonymous*. We return home and review our work on the first Five Steps.

- We consider the *foundation* of complete willingness (*AA* 12). Am I willing to go to any length for my recovery?

- We consider the *cement* of our common problem and our common solution (*AA* 17). Do I believe I am powerless over lust? Do I accept the SA program as my Higher Power's solution for me? Am I willing to work the remaining Steps in order to grow into the person my Higher Power would have me be?

- We consider the *cornerstone* of belief in a Higher Power. "Do I now believe, or am I even willing to believe, that there is a Power greater than myself?" (*AA* 47). Am I willing to let go of my unhealthy ideas about God?

- We consider the *keystone* of not taking charge (*AA* 62). Am I willing to quit playing God? Am I willing to surrender my will and my life to the care of God as I understand God? Am I willing to follow rather than lead? Am I willing to accept Good Orderly Direction from others in the program? Do I admit the folly of self-will?

We prayerfully ask if we have omitted anything and whether our Step work is solid so far. We share this review with our sponsor. Some of us find it helpful to share briefly the results of this review at our next SA meeting. When we are satisfied with our work, we are ready for Step Six.

## *Some Questions to Consider*

1. Did the cautionary remarks on page 74 in *Alcoholics Anonymous* affect my decision about who should hear my inventory? How?

2. What is the difference between sharing my inventory with God and with another human being?

3. What is the risk of admitting the exact nature of my wrongs to another person?

4. How did I benefit from sharing things I had planned to keep secret?

5. What have I learned about the exact nature of my wrongs?

6. If I later remember events or persons who ought to have been part of my Fifth Step but were not, what will I do?

7. How has Step Five changed my perception of myself?

# *Step Six*

## *Were entirely ready to have God remove all these defects of character*

Our work on the Steps so far showed us that we had to change if we were to live a useful, meaningful life. Our physical, mental, emotional, and spiritual health depended on that change. If we could have changed on our own, we would have done it long ago. We realized that we would not be able to remove our own defects of character. Our part was to be ready to change; God would provide the power in our lives.

We needed a different attitude from the old pleading that some of us did with God: "Help me stop acting out!" or "Save me from my jealousy!" or "Don't let me rage again!" In those prayers our self-will was looking for a magical answer. We were looking for rescue, not recovery. We wanted instant relief rather than a change of mind and heart. Step Six was where we became ready to let go of self-will and old patterns of behavior. Our new perspective came from the work we had done on the first five Steps.

> By now the newcomer has probably arrived at the following conclusions: that his character defects, representing instincts gone astray, have been the primary cause of his [lusting] and his failure at life; that unless he is now willing to work hard at the elimination of the worst of these defects, both sobriety and peace of mind will still elude him; that all the faulty foundation of his life will have to be torn out and built anew on bedrock.
> (*12&12* 50)

We found that we were powerless over our character defects in the same way that we were powerless over lust. Although we were powerless, because we now had a relationship with a Power greater than ourselves, we were not helpless. If we could be granted freedom from lust, could we not also be freed from our character defects? Step Six required that we do everything within our power to forsake our defects and begin to trust that God would handle their removal. We began a lifelong process of watching for our character defects to arise, doing what we could to correct them, and becoming willing to have them removed. We became willing through a process: prayer that we would be made aware of our shortcomings, eventual acceptance of our powerlessness over them, willingness to have them removed, and a growing faith that our Higher Power could change us.

Sometimes we were not ready to let go of certain character defects. We have said, "Please remove my rage." On reflection, however, we realized that letting go of rage might not be possible without also surrendering our judgment of ourselves and others. We then added: "But I'm not ready to have that removed yet." The key word here is *yet*. If we were completely unwilling, we found that there were consequences such as pain, desperation, continuing our double life, and loss of our sobriety. As long as we could see the possibility of becoming willing, we were still in the program. At times of unwillingness, we prayed for willingness.

When we willfully went against our conscience, our disease was ready and waiting to become the center of our life again. This was not punishment; it was consequence, a natural law of cause and effect. As our intention shifted toward working in harmony with life and contributing to it, we began to accept and learn from the consequences of our choices. We also began to realize we could ask for help and work the Program to avoid further pain to ourselves and others.

We applied Step Six wherever we wanted change to occur in ourselves. We found that our freedom was based on daily acceptance of our character defects. Although they tended to pop up anew every day, this was not necessarily a bad thing—this was part of being human. We would always need a Power greater than ourselves in our lives. Each day, we needed that Power to remove those defects that fed our insanity and blocked us from God and from others. Step Six asked that we be willing to change and be changed. Although we may have initially wanted all our defects eliminated, many of us came to the realization that our defects can teach us humility and wisdom.

We saw that what appeared to be a character defect in one situation could be an asset in another. We realized that some of these defects were actually good character traits that we had misused, "instincts gone astray" (*12&12* 50). We had taken discretion to the extreme of harsh judgment, conscientiousness to the extreme of perfectionism, concern for the opinion of others to the extreme of dependency on their approval. Step Six gave us the humility to allow our Higher Power to use all of our character traits for a greater good. Through working the Steps, we gained insight that allowed us a new understanding of our character. We saw how we could accept and value ourselves even in our brokenness. God could use us—defects and all —if we just continue seeking to become the person He wants us to be.

## *Members of SA Share*

*1*

Step Six works for me one defect at a time. I don't think anyone really expects to have their shortcomings removed all at once. That would be too much of a shock to one's system, not to mention family and friends. So I take my character defects one at a time, as they arise, and surrender them. I find that as I become willing to admit I'm wrong or to make more amends, I become willing to surrender more defects.

*2*

After completing Step Five with my sponsor I had great hope and high energy for my program. Up to that point surrender had always meant doing something. For example, I surrendered my isolation by showing up at meetings, speaking up, making phone calls, and getting a sponsor. I always found God asking me to take positive steps on faith to surrender my right to give in to my disease. But now God was asking me simply to "get ready" to surrender my defects. Suddenly, all my goal-oriented activity came to a screeching halt and I was left standing there becoming entirely ready.

I discovered that my overly competitive, compulsive drives

were slowly dying and being replaced by the hunger for God that they had been covering up my whole life. I was beginning to learn to wait on God. The first Five Steps had taught me how to use the Program to surrender my sickness—vital skills that I still call upon daily and sometimes hourly—but now I was beginning to learn to surrender even my program to God. I had made the decision to turn my will and my life over in Step Three, but now I was learning what that meant on the inside. The black hole that Step Six had been for me was gradually being transformed by God into one more building block in my life foundation. I was learning to rely on the principle of becoming entirely ready as I move through all the Steps. For me, Step Six is a truth that I now try to practice every day as God gives me the strength.

*3*

I reluctantly admitted I had a problem that I could not handle myself (Step One). I knew I needed the help of a "Professional" (Step Two). I decided to put myself in the hands of a Power greater than myself (Step Three). I then had to face the pain my addiction has caused for me and those I love (Step Four), acknowledging the decay in my life and confessing it to someone else (Step Five).

It was like admitting I have a tooth problem, deciding to make an appointment, and having it x-rayed. If the picture shows the tooth is clearly rotten, it needs to come out. Until I become willing to make the next appointment, nothing will change for the better. In fact, it will eventually get worse and poison me.

My inventory has shown me exactly where the rottenness exists. I have gazed into the "cavity," rigorously admitted the truth, and must make a decision. I can continue to trust my own will in an attempt to deny or change the past or to maintain control. Or instead, I can recognize the operation of a Higher Power who is waiting to extract the painful decay, bringing me out of the past and into the present. Only then can I begin to turn away from my obsession with self and turn toward greater usefulness to God and others.

*4*

For me, a practical insight in Step Six came with the understanding of the word *remove.* I always thought that if God were to remove my defects of character they would be obliterated, destroyed, erased—never to return. Wrong! Remove is one of those words like re-member, re-union, or re-connect. "*Re*" comes from the Latin root meaning "to do again."

By working all of the Steps, God has moved my glaring personality flaws from where they are quite visible to a place where they are not so obvious. Are they still there? You bet! All I have to add is a little self-will, and they come screaming back to the forefront of my behavior. They will inflict all kinds of havoc on me and on those around me. If I am willing to have God remove these defects of character, I am assured that God will lead me to a better life.

*5*

My Creator gave me instincts for a purpose. When I let these instincts exceed the purpose for which they are intended, they cause problems. When I imagine God ripping these instincts from me in some sort of brutal psychological surgery, I fear being left with gaping wounds where my instincts used to be. Instead of this frightening image, I think of these instincts gone astray as a compass that is a few degrees off true. If I use this compass to fly from New York to Los Angeles, the few degrees of error over the length of my trip may send me to Mexico. Similarly, pursuing instincts that are off the mark of God's intended purpose leads me away from my intended goal. In becoming entirely ready to have God remove these defects, I am actually becoming ready for Him to realign my compass and bring my instincts back into line with His will for me. I am becoming ready for Him to restore me to sanity.

*6*

I was recently thinking of my attitude about fear. As an adult I have hated my fear because it keeps me boxed-in and unwilling to make changes and move forward. Then I realized that this attitude is not completely honest. I know better than that. It was fear that got me into recovery. It was fear that kept me from hurting people even more than I did. It was fear that sent me to college. It was fear that kept me in relationships. I could go on all night about what fear has done. The point is that not all my fear is bad. It gets bad when it keeps me from growing spiritually.

As a result, I can look on fear as an old friend, a motivator that I really needed at one time but don't need much anymore. I don't need to hate this emotion because, at times, it has served a good purpose. When I had no trust or faith, I needed fear to keep me going. Now, however, I need to start using fear less and using trust and faith more. I think this is what Step Six is all about.

7

When I first came to SA, I just wanted to stop a few clearly self-destructive behaviors. I bought into the whole "lust" deal; I wanted to stop that too. So, after getting sober and being relieved of those major "bad habits," I felt I was good enough. Can't I just coast along? God, could you maybe leave me alone now and let me do my thing? As a sponsee of mine later said, "I don't want to be a monk. I just want to be a good guy." (He subsequently left the program and went back out there.)

SA and the God of my understanding don't work that way. For an addict like me, it has to be all or nothing. Half-measures do not result in lasting sobriety or recovery. In Step Three, I turn my will and my life over to a Higher Power—not the bad parts of my will or the parts of my life related to my sexaholism. My will and life. *All* my thoughts and *all* my behaviors. Everything I am and everything I have. Everything I will ever be and everything I will ever have. God as I understand Him doesn't want an hour a week for a meeting; He doesn't want my defects; He doesn't want my time in service to Him or my fellows. He wants me. The Program of SA is about surrendering myself more and more to Him, progressively shedding all of my character defects, seeking his perfect ideals. That's what I am in for—that's the price of recovery. That is what SA and the God I came to know offer. Nothing less.

Initially I couldn't see that there really is no better path than this "Road of Happy Destiny." I didn't think peace and joy could compare to the excitement and passion that had been the focus of my life for so long. Wow, I was never more wrong about anything! Recovery—working the SA Program—is a far better life than I could ever imagine back then. I have a long way to go; but, over the years, I have seen God slowly, painfully lead me towards who He wants me to be. There is only one power in the universe that can stop Him from succeeding: me, if I choose lust over Him. I choose recovery.

*8*

One of the ways that I have grown to work Step Six is to use the items in my pockets as symbols of portions of my life that I do not want to surrender. For instance, a chain of keys represents my dishonest illusion that I am actually in control. A wallet represents my fear of financial insecurity and self-centered lust for more stuff. A pager and a name badge represent the unrealistic expectations that I and others have of me at work. A cell phone represents my relationships with others, which I have often manipulated to get what I want. Sometimes during prayer I clean my pockets out as an act of willingness. At night, if I have particularly struggled with a certain defect or area of life, I choose the object in my pockets that most represents that area, and I let it lie overnight on a table that I have turned into a small altar to my Higher Power.

*9*

In approaching this Step, it helps me to look at my defects of character in the same way that I looked at the lust that continued after I began to surrender my acting out. I didn't encounter the force of my lust until I stopped the acting out. Similarly, I couldn't see how much power my defects of character had over me until I saw, in my Fourth and Fifth Steps, how they almost destroyed me.

I find myself returning to Step Six because my defects, like my lust, are always there. If left untreated, they can lead me back to acting out. I deal with the defects as I deal with lust, primarily by identifying them (self-centeredness, procrastination, dishonesty) and by being accountable to others in my willingness to let God remove them. As with lust, the temptation is there, but I don't have to act on it.

*10*

When I first read Step Six, I didn't think it made much sense. It seemed superfluous. I thought maybe Bill W. just didn't like having eleven Steps, so he added this one because twelve sounded better than eleven. In *Alcoholics Anonymous*, there are only two paragraphs on Step Six, which appears to suggest we spend only one hour on it! However, in *Twelve Steps and Twelve Traditions*, we are told that this is the Step that "separates the men from the boys." It is possibly the most important Step!

This reflects my personal experience. Over the years, the importance of Step Six has become more and more evident to me. At one time, in our area, our meetings were heavily focused on Steps Four and Five. We saw that many members were stuck on Step Four, so we had a sponsor workshop and helped encourage everyone to complete their inventories. We got very good at writing inventories. However, as the weeks and months passed, we noticed many people continuing to share the same life struggles in meeting after meeting. It became obvious that an inventory of our character defects—even a good thorough one that is shared with our sponsor—isn't enough. Knowing my defects doesn't make my life any better; I have to actually give them up. That's why Steps Six and Seven are so important.

## *Step into Action*

### *Recommended Readings*

We suggest that members read and study the following before working the Step:

*Alcoholics Anonymous* (*AA*)
"Into Action" 76

*Sexaholics Anonymous* (*SA*)
"Steps Six and Seven" 115-121

*Twelve Steps and Twelve Traditions* (*12&12*)
"Step Six" 63-69

## *One Method for Working Step Six*

We believe that practicing Step Six is a lifelong process. Yet we should not be distracted or delayed from moving forward to Steps Seven, Eight, and Nine. Just as we practiced Steps Two and Three by working Step Four, part of practicing Steps Six and Seven is moving on to the subsequent Steps. *Alcoholics Anonymous* (76) describes Step Six as an assessment of our attitude before we begin the Seventh Step Prayer. Are we willing? If not, we pray for willingness. We are not given a time frame, but the text implies only momentary reflection.

One way we become ready to have our shortcomings removed is to admit them to other sober members of the Fellowship. We admit our powerlessness and our state of readiness to have our shortcomings removed. Some of us find the following Step Six exercise helpful. It can be used any time we are having trouble surrendering a shortcoming. This exercise also helps us identify ways to put some positive alternatives into action in our daily lives.

We write the exercise in a spiral notebook. First we list the most destructive character defects or patterns of behavior that we and our sponsor identified during our Fifth Step. We then turn the page to have two blank facing pages on which to write. There are four columns, two to a page.

We label the far left column on the left page "Defects." Here we place the first character defect from our list. Sometimes we perceive these defects as operating separately, sometimes we see them operating in pairs or clusters. We list them as we see them in our lives. The rest of the left page is the second column. We label it "Life with this defect." Here, we describe how this defect affects our lives. How does this defect affect our relationships with others and with ourselves? What does this behavior cost us and others? What payoffs or benefits do we think we are receiving? What feelings do we associate with this behavior in the moment or later in reflection? What patterns trigger this defect or are triggered by this defect? What do we fear losing by letting go of this character defect? Most of the right page is for the third column, labeled "Vision of life without this defect." Here we describe our vision of how our lives might be if we were completely free of this shortcoming. What alternative behaviors might we practice instead? What is the opposite of this defect? What might we gain by surrendering it? How might the quality of our lives improve? How might we be different in our relationships and at work? How might removal of this defect affect our productivity, serenity, and usefulness to others? How might our relationship with the God of our understanding grow?

Seeing, in black and white, the difference between life as we know it and the vision of life without this problem is often the motivation we need to spark our willingness to let go of this defect of character. Some of us write a goodbye letter to our shortcoming, thanking it for helping us cope and telling it we don't need it anymore.

Extracting the essence of this vision in the form of a prayer is useful as a way to carry this vision and willingness with us and to reinforce it on a regular basis. We can repeat this prayer every time we see that particular defect manifesting in some way. We label the fourth column "My Prayer." These short, simple prayers support our willingness to surrender these defects to the God of our understanding. Our sponsor often helps us write these. Some of us use these prayers daily and carry them with us on a card.

We repeat this procedure for each character defect on our list. When we share this work with our sponsor and notice the dramatic difference between life *with* and life *without* each character defect, we become more and more willing to surrender them – we become more and more ready for the new life. We are ready to move on to Step Seven.

Here are two examples of a Sixth Step exercise:

| *Defect* | *Life with this defect* | *Vision of life without this defect* | *My Prayer* |
|---|---|---|---|
| Poor self-esteem | I avoid people, social situations, and talking on the phone.<br><br>I avoid honestly expressing my opinions.<br><br>I see myself as impatient, controlling, and demanding.<br><br>I have an unhealthy dependence on others.<br><br>I cling to the idea that at least I am not totally alone.<br><br>I violate my own values and lose self-respect. | I would welcome social interaction as an opportunity to serve and love God and others.<br><br>I would see myself as a spiritual being on a path of growth, service, and peace.<br><br>I would pursue the approval of my God and begin to discover who God wants me to be.<br><br>I would make friends with those who accept and appreciate me.<br><br>I would be true to my values. | "God, help me to be the kind and compassionate person you want me to be.<br><br>"Help me to continue to be a good and generous friend.<br><br>"Allow me to better see the gifts you have already provided and to be grateful for the progress you have made in me."<br><br>"God, thank you for loving me in spite of my remaining defects!<br><br>"Help me to remember that my worth comes from being your child and not from what other people think of me.<br><br>"Let me continue to seek to please you, instead of trying to please others." |

## *Some Questions to Consider*

1. How has working Steps One through Five provided a strong foundation for the remaining Steps?
2. While sharing Step Five with another human being, what patterns of behavior did I uncover that led to lust, resentments, or fear?
3. Did I identify behavior patterns or character defects that I am not yet ready to have removed? What are my fears about letting them go?
4. What does "entirely ready" mean to me? Why will I need courage to become entirely ready?
5. What are the differences and similarities between my lust or sexual addiction and my defects of character?
6. How would I describe my discovery, growing awareness, and surrender of my character defects?

# *Step Seven*

## *Humbly asked Him to remove our shortcomings*

Step Seven requires humility. Humility is honest, accurate self-perception. Humility is seeing ourselves right-sized, rightly proportioned to our Higher Power and our fellows. Humility is seeing ourselves as we really are, as our Higher Power would see us. *Twelve Steps and Twelve Traditions* defines humility as "a clear recognition of what and who we really are, followed by a sincere attempt to become what we could be. Therefore, our first practical move toward humility must consist of recognizing our deficiencies. No defect can be corrected unless we clearly see what it is (*12&12* 58). Thinking highly or lowly of ourselves is a form of pride or fear, and humility is the opposite of both.

Humility means:

- We recognize our own powerlessness over the situation.
- We have surrendered and let go of our attachment to the result.
- We know that we need to *ask* because we are not the ones with the answers.
- We are willing to be taught and to do our part.
- We are entirely ready.
- We desire to seek and do God's will.

Before recovery, we knew little of humility. We concerned ourselves with our own lusts and desires. If only we could gain wealth, romance, or success, *then* we could be modest about it. Many of us saw achieving, possessing, and acquiring as the means to happiness and as the purpose of our lives. In an endless cycle of dissatisfaction, we sought to serve ourselves. Real spiritual growth and character development were not priorities, indeed were not even possible in that state. We lived life as a tribute to our desires and our dependencies. Our pride, sometimes disguised as shame and self-condemnation, obscured who we really were. Pride was one of the activators of our "dis-ease."

As long as we lacked a relationship with a Power greater than ourselves, we were masquerading as that power, and we could not know humility. As long as we were running the show, our self-will brought misery. Through working the Steps, we began to see that we were absolutely dependent on a Power greater than ourselves for our recovery and our lives. As we continued to surrender more of ourselves to the will of our Creator, we found happiness, joy, and freedom. As we grew in humility we grew in sobriety and usefulness to others.

As we read Step Seven we wondered how we could learn to be humble. Then we recognized that we had learned something of humility while working the previous Steps. We already had surrendered our fear and pride in telling our sponsor and group about our history and our powerlessness. In meetings, we continued to be honest about our struggles, regardless of what others thought of us. In order to stay sober and to make progress in the Steps,

> We ask God to remove our defects, but we start taking the actions required, for "Faith without action is dead." On a daily, hourly, moment-by-moment basis we begin. Usually it's one defect at a time, every time it shows up. One incident, one encounter, one trial at a time, we stop, look, and listen to our feelings and review what happened. Sometimes we have to write it out to see it. No matter what wrong the other party has done, *if we are disturbed, there is always something wrong with us* (*SA* 116-117).

Our task was to learn to see ourselves realistically, not as we wanted to appear. Each Step had helped us by requiring that we relinquish pieces of the old self-image we had created. Also, we had to strive for a "manner of living which demands rigorous honesty" (*AA* 58).

At first we saw that we were out of control. We needed the Steps to show us how to let go of our delusions of self-sufficiency.

Admitting that we weren't up to the task of managing our life, we were ready for help and direction from God. We came to believe that, though broken, we were worthy of this help. We became willing to be guided and to be taught. We acknowledged things about ourselves that we never wanted to admit. As we brought our character flaws into the light, we saw that we were human and recognized the futility of trying to convince ourselves that we had to be perfect in order to be worthwhile. We came to accept our inability to change on our own, yet we believed we could be changed and could be of service. As we discovered the truth about ourselves, we were learning a true sense of humility. We saw that the path to spiritual growth was to continue working the Steps.

Like humility, the process of asking was unfamiliar to us. Before recovery we had demanded, cajoled, pleaded, dreamed, negotiated, manipulated, or lusted to get what we wanted. Step Seven required that we turn to a Source greater than ourselves and ask for what we wanted. With our changed attitude, we asked without expectation. We trusted that our Higher Power would give us what we needed, although it might not be what we wanted. When we asked humbly, we acknowledged that we didn't know what was best for us. We might not understand the answers, and we might not even recognize them as answers. We might not understand the implications of what we were asking for. We asked humbly, without an agenda, without an ulterior motive, without attachment to the result.

Perfectionism is a character defect; but, paradoxically, striving for moral perfection is what the Steps asked of us. We had to recognize that it is impossible to achieve, and that we could only grow in that direction with the aid of our Higher Power. We would never get there in our lifetime, but it had to be our goal. Striving for moral perfection, but accepting that we wouldn't be perfect, is part of humility.

When we asked for our shortcomings to be removed, we were asking that we be brought to a place where we could begin to be contributing members of a society of peers. We had made it our habit to be takers, but we wanted to change. We believed that God's will for us and the path to true happiness was to become useful members of our groups, our families, and our communities.

Step Seven taught us to live with a degree of uncertainty. This uncertainty helped us to surrender the idea that we could control life and make it work out the way we wanted. We trusted that our Higher Power really is in control and has our best interests at heart. We were prepared to receive something other than what we asked for. We were being taught to live life in a way we had never accepted before. Perhaps our view of our defects was not helpful. Perhaps some of our defects would turn out to be useful. We would let God decide how we could be useful to others. We didn't know what life might look like after removal of a shortcoming. We didn't know how long it might take, or how removal might be accomplished. We gave up judging ourselves when we didn't meet our own standards. We became teachable. The Steps had been asking us progressively to give up our agendas and our ideas of how we thought life should be. Step Seven brought us to the deepest surrender thus far.

Humbly asking, we began to leave our self-centeredness behind. This took time. We gradually became more aware of our Higher Power's bidding. As we became willing to follow, our shortcomings became less of an impediment. Asking without expectation left us in a place of acceptance. We let go of the results. We found ourselves back in the present moment, ready to take care of what was in front of us. The problem—those shortcomings we had identified in previous Steps—was in better hands.

When ready to let them go, we ask God to give us the power to overcome them. We need to clean up our side of the street, to make our amends, and to complete Steps Eight and Nine. We practiced Step Seven to align our will with God's will as we went out into the world. We experienced the serenity of being in the solution.

> *Victory through powerlessness by the grace of God!*
> That's the beautiful paradox of this program: In and through my powerlessness, I receive the power—and love—that come from above.

Acknowledging what I am, surrendering, and relying on God's power bring release, freedom, and joy.
Recovery is an inside job (*SA* 168).

## *Members of SA Share*

*1*

One way I approached the Seventh Step was to take my list of character defects and put together a personal Seventh Step prayer based upon my own faith tradition and the God of my understanding. Here is what I came up with:

- Thank You for meeting me at the point of my need.
- To You who are perfectly humble, I give my pride.
- To You who support all of creation by Your diligence, I give my laziness.
- To You who stand ready to forgive all, I give my resent-ment.
- To You who are without guilt and beyond reproach, I give my shame.
- To You who do not flinch, I surrender all my fear and timidity.
- To You the Creator who needs nothing, I give all my spiritual, emotional, and physical neediness.
- To You who are all giving, I give my greed.
- To You who are eternally patient, I give my impatience.
- To You who are worthy of complete trust, I give my doubt.
- I trust You to give me what I need because You are You.

Once I identified and surrendered my powerlessness over lust, I was in a position to address my character defects. As much as my lust ever did, it is these defects that stand in the way of my usefulness to God and my fellows. Even though I have not acted out in years, Step Seven reminds me that I am still a broken person, but with hope for a better future of useful service and spiritual growth.

*2*

My character defects are removed for one day. The next day these defects may come back bigger than the day before, but I have learned to use the tools of the program. If I don't take the actions I took yesterday, I may not have another day of serenity. And for me this program is about comfort—being comfortable in my own skin.

*3*

Before working the Steps, I thought humble meant humiliated. To me it meant feeling *less than*, embarrassed, angry—the way I felt in the judgmental environment of my youth. Humility meant being abused by a disrespectful power greater than myself. I thought it described an uncomfortable situation where I lost my self-respect. I thought that if a task were too big for me, I was too small to be worthwhile. I thought I was less than I should be: that there was something wrong with me.

Working the Steps helped me see that it was okay to be me. There were many things I couldn't do under my own power; that was not only okay, but it was the way things worked and the way it was supposed to be. I learned that humility means seeing things as they really are. Many things in life really are too big for me. I need to rely on a Power greater than myself, and I need to be open to learning.

This gift of humility that I got from working the Steps, that I try to practice one day at a time, frees me to be who I am, rather than who I think I should be. I am a person who has strengths, weaknesses, likes, dislikes, and desires. I am worthwhile and worthy of respect because I am a person.

My Higher Power is willing to teach me to see the world in a different way and to make me useful. I only have to ask.

*4*

I just pulled a dog-eared list of my character defects out of my wallet. The top two items on this list are pride and self-righteousness. I have prayed to God that they be removed. Yet today's inventory finds them still active, in particular with attitudes and behaviors toward my wife. Before getting down on myself because these are still active many years after first taking Step Seven, I want to make sure my inventory is thorough.

Is this really the same pride and self-righteousness that I first looked at many years ago? I don't think so. I was very comfortable with my conceits for years. But now, even when I compulsively indulge them, they are no longer comfortable conceits. Perhaps the pain and discomfort I now feel is God slowly, carefully, and graciously doing for me what I could not do for myself.

I had thought I was entirely ready to have these defects removed, but God knows me much better than I do. Today's pain is not a constant pain. I do get reprieves. There are days when the promises seem right at my fingertips; freedom from pride and self-righteousness seems almost as real as freedom from lust can often be for me. Fretting over whether or not God has removed *all* my pride and self-righteousness is focusing on the problem. I need only be entirely ready to have God remove *today's* defects.

*5*

My inability to complete Steps Six and Seven in AA is what got me to take Step One in SA. I was not entirely ready to have God remove all my defects of character. Free from alcohol, I did not want to stop acting out sexually, and I knew that without completing my Step work, I could not retain my alcohol abstinence. One day after leaving a porno shop in utter hopelessness, I met the person who told me about SA. He invited me to my first SA meeting. I was ready that day.

It was just the two of us at that first meeting. Since that day many years ago, I have experienced the miracle of sobriety.

My character defects are taking their time to leave. There is greed, there is envy, and there is control—to mention a few. The miracle is that they are lessening, and at least I am usually aware of them when they appear. My sponsor tells me that I am better than I used to be but not as well as I am going to get.

*6*

I wanted to hear from people who had a lot of experience in working the Steps, so I started attending an AA Step Study meeting. At the first meeting there were about 25 people, with more than 450 years of sobriety among them. The topic was "Humbly asked Him to remove our shortcomings."

Almost the entire meeting was taken up discussing the first word: humbly. With my one week of sobriety, I was in awe of these people. Even those with 15, 20, 25, and 39 years of sobriety were all talking about humility. These fine folks with decades of recovery were talking from their heart and from their daily experiences of how humility had helped their recovery. And to top it off, they were talking about their gratitude for the humility they had gained in working the Steps.

That was strong medicine for this sick newcomer. The idea of humility was etched into my brain. I came to believe that these Twelve Step folks truly walked their talk and that they had what I wanted. I try to carry the lesson of the practical importance of humility with me today.

*7*

For me, humility is a place where I can go inside myself. It's a mixture of awe, a connection with God and other people, and gratitude that doesn't have to be expressed. It means joy and peace at the same time. Nothing can get to me when I'm in this space. Sometimes it lasts only a few moments, but it is there. I never would have thought that such a gift would come from facing my character defects.

*8*

More than any other Step, Step Seven deals with my motives in all of my interactions with others. In my acting out days, I believed that if I appeared honest and moral on the job, this would help me to get what I wanted. But in recovery, it is suggested that I practice these principles without expectation of reward, simply because it is the right thing to do. If I'm working the program, I don't engage in *displays* of honesty, I *become* honest. I don't just talk about the virtues of open-mindedness; I actually start to listen to others, first in my home group, then at home and on the job. Then, one day at a time, I let go of ego-driven plans and agendas, regardless of what it might cost me or how this might appear to others.

I also must avoid inventing a spiritual motive when I secretly want to get my own way. I need to check my motives in volunteering for, or avoiding, certain service positions. The good news is, if I participate to the best of my ability in all aspects of the program, interacting wholeheartedly and honestly with others at business meetings, in sponsorship, and service, I can't help but grow in genuine humility. I have witnessed the lessening of the power of my defects by a loving God.

*9*

I live a sober life by God's grace. I accept that sexual sobriety alone does not guarantee healing. It makes healing possible because it allows God to enter into and change my life. Just as sobriety is a gift from God, God's progressive healing of my defective nature is also a gift.

I humbly ask God to remove my shortcomings because He has proven that He will, just as He removes my compulsion to act out in lust. I humbly ask God to remove my shortcomings because He knows better than I do what is best for me. Though I find myself continually falling short of God's will, He is able to bridge the gap. He changes what others hear in my words so that what I share is still helpful, even though I am imperfect.

*10*

I believe honesty is the key to humility. I developed a nodding acquaintance with humility when I wrote out my First Step and shared it with my sponsor. I took another step toward humility when I shared my story with my home group and listened to the feedback of other members. I took a further step in humility when I wrote out my Fourth Step and shared it with my sponsor. All of this didn't happen overnight or in a logical or sequential way. It took a process of willingness coupled with action spread over months and years. This process is still going on.

To grow in humility, I have to practice the principles of the Program in all of my affairs. Am I honest on my resume and in my tax returns? Am I considerate and careful while driving? Am I always willing to be absolutely honest with God, myself, and others in the Fellowship about where I'm failing to measure up, particularly in my lust recovery? Am I hiding behind the badge of my calendar sobriety? All this tells me that true humility doesn't come easily for a recovering sexaholic, but it does come if I'm prepared to practice honesty.

*11*

For me, willingness was the key to this Step. The knob was on my side of the door. As I opened the door a crack, the grace of God poured into my life, like sunlight into the darkness of a dungeon. Self-reliance had failed me miserably, but reliance on God brought me into a successful way of living.

## *Step into Action*

### *Recommended Readings*

We suggest that members read and study the following before working the Step:

*Alcoholics Anonymous* (*AA*)
"Into Action" 76

*Sexaholics Anonymous* (*SA*)
"Steps Six and Seven" 115-121

*Twelve Steps and Twelve Traditions* (*12&12*)
"Step Seven" 70-76

## *One Method for Working Step Seven*

Based on our moral inventory we have a list of character defects. We ask ourselves whether we are ready to have God remove all of these. If not, we pray for willingness. With all our heart and soul, we open ourselves to our Creator and ask for help. In asking, many of us use AA's Seventh Step prayer.

> My Creator, I am now willing that you should have all of me, good and bad. I pray that you now remove from me every single defect of character which stands in the way of my usefulness to you and my fellows. Grant me strength, as I go out from here, to do your bidding. Amen (*AA* 76).

These words express a new relationship with our Higher Power. The tone is different from the Third Step prayer, reflecting the work we have done in Steps Four through Six and our recognition that God has helped us to do that work. We sit with, or phone, our sponsors and repeat this prayer, thus completing Step Seven.

Like the rest of the Steps, we use Step Seven every day. We practice humility daily, asking our Higher Power to guide us and change us. In Step Six we accept our imperfections and our powerlessness over them but learn to surrender our shortcomings and affirm our desire for improvement. In Step Seven we take that attitude and awareness into prayer. We renew our surrender and ask to be made useful to others, to do the right thing, to do our Higher Power's bidding. We let go of the results of this prayer and our desire to control them. We often find that we must practice this many times each day. We keep a list of our defects with us. We carry it around and work on it at least once daily.

While many of us use the Seventh Step prayer from *Alcoholics Anonymous*, some of us write our own personal versions of the Seventh Step prayer. These may relate to our own faith tradition or to our own personal understanding of our Higher Power. Some of us pray repeatedly over specific shortcomings and eventually we do become willing to let go of our old behaviors.

We use Step Seven whenever we are ready to have one of our

shortcomings removed. Some of us review our character defects daily and ask God to remove them. We don't expect that the result will be accomplished without our participation. God will remove our dishonesty, but we must practice being honest. When we ask for patience, God gives us opportunities to practice patience. God will remove our self-centeredness, but we must practice taking the actions of love to help others while we are waiting. We can do something positive in place of a shortcoming, like practicing the opposite behavior. Many of us find that regular practice of these 'opposite behaviors' is an essential part of having our defects removed. In simple but profound words, the whole program can be reduced to what someone discovered for himself: "Without God, I can't; Without me, God won't" (*SA* 96).

Carrying Step Seven with us every day as an attitude means that while we are aware of our shortcomings, we are not obsessed with their removal or with managing them ourselves. We are content to constantly turn them over and trust that they will be changed the way they need to be. We recognize that our defects are rooted in our being. For their removal we must depend on and cooperate with our Higher Power, doing our best to clean up our side of the street and keep it clean. All the while we watch for what our Higher Power would teach us, reminding ourselves we are no longer in charge.

The humble attitude of Step Seven allows God to move us toward forgiving ourselves and others. Then we move on to work Steps Eight and Nine.

## *Some Questions to Consider*

1. What character traits or beliefs block my ability to be humble?

2. What does being humble mean to me? How has someone I know demonstrated humility?

3. What fears do I have about working Step Seven? How might giving up my defects of character change my personality?

4. Which character defect interferes most with my recovery today? How willing am I to ask my Higher Power to remove it? Is there a specific action I need to take that I am avoiding?

5. What happens when I trust my Higher Power to remove my defects of character?

6. How has humility changed my view of myself and my character while working the Steps?

7. How have I become teachable?

8. What gifts might I receive as my Higher Power removes my shortcomings?

9. What does "Humbly asked Him to remove our shortcomings" mean to you?

## *Step Eight*

### *Made a list of all persons we had harmed, and became willing to make amends to them all*

Some of us put off Step Eight because we were fearful of the amends called for in Step Nine. In effect, we were trying to manage tomorrow instead of living in today. We soon realized, however, that we ought to fear the consequences of *not* working Step Eight (such as remaining a prisoner to our guilt and shame), so we surrendered our self-centered fears and took the necessary action.

Some of us were convinced that people on our amends list actually owed *us* amends and used this as an excuse for delaying. Harboring resentment or keeping score would actually nourish our craving for lust and short-circuit our recovery. Step Eight told us to focus on the harm we had done and become willing to make amends for that. We could not wish or will the guilt away. Only when we stopped running, when we turned around and looked them full in the face and set about making them right, was their power over us broken. That's when we were set free (*SA* 123).

Others felt that our past misdeeds were unforgivable, and we rationalized that making amends would be pointless and shaming, or dangerous to others or ourselves. But as we prayed for forgiveness and practiced acceptance of ourselves, we realized that believing we were unforgivable was one of the lies we told ourselves. One benefit of making amends, we discovered, was our ability to identify and correct these lies. Persisting in the belief that we were unforgivable was really prideful and grandiose. Making mistakes, even those that caused harm to others, brought us opportunities to learn and grow. We began to accept ourselves and others as people who make mistakes and do harm from time to time. We found that we could experience release from guilt and remorse.

The shortcomings that kept us from working Step Eight were the same as those we had become ready to have God remove in Step Six and humbly asked Him to remove in Step Seven. In Step

Eight, we simply turned the results of that process over to God and did the next right thing that was in front of us.

We put our trust in God and followed the direction of our sponsor and others who had benefited by taking these Steps. We prayed for willingness and found that our fears began to diminish as soon as we took the action of writing our list. Often we began with names from our Fourth Step inventory. Then we added others we may have forgotten about, as well as those less directly affected by our behavior. We saw that the harm we caused sometimes had far-reaching effects. Writing a list of *all* those we had harmed showed us the unrecognized consequences of our behavior.

We also realized that forgiving ourselves and others was essential to the process of making amends. As *Sexaholics Anonymous* (125) advises, "Somewhere between making the list and making the amends, there's an unwritten requirement that we forgive. (Although there seem to be times when we have to make the amends *before* we can forgive)." If we could not forgive, then we remained chained to our resentments, and our recovery was thwarted. If we didn't feel forgiving, we simply took the actions of forgiving and prayed that God would change our heart.

For each entry on our Step Eight list, we prayerfully considered how we had harmed the individual and how we could make amends. As in other areas of our recovery, we discovered it was hazardous to make amends without guidance from our sponsor and people who had already worked these Steps. Selfishness and rationalization might distract us or cause us to adopt the attitude that we had never hurt anyone but ourselves.

Why forgive? For us it is very simple. If we don't forgive, we're never free. Unless we forgive, we are not forgiven; we remain chained to our wrongs, unable to free ourselves, leave the dark dungeon of our past, and walk in the sunlight of love (*SA* 126). This attitude, of course, is the end result of purposeful forgetting. It is an attitude which can only be changed by a deep and honest search of our motives and actions (*12&12* 79).

Our goal in Step Eight was to *become willing* to make amends to those we had harmed, regardless of whether we anticipated that the other person would accept our amends and regardless of whether we anticipated actually being able to make direct amends.

We worked Step Eight to ensure continued progress in recovery and lasting sobriety. As we faced our past and became willing to correct what we could, we opened ourselves further to a humble relationship with a Power greater than ourselves. It is that Power who would provide the opportunities for us to right our wrongs in Step Nine.

## *Members of SA Share*

*1*

I was afraid to make a list. I wanted to take the Fifth Amendment to avoid incriminating myself! Without knowing it, I had cornered myself with the unconscious belief that I had harmed *everyone*, and that I was too bad to be worthy of the new life that recovery offered. When I couldn't avoid it any longer and actually wrote the list, I was surprised at the relief. My list was finite.

*2*

As I approached Step Eight, I ran into a roadblock of personal pride: I believed that the wrongs I did and the mistakes I made were unforgivable, so I thought amends were impossible. How could I forgive others if I could not forgive myself? As I worked Step Eight, I asked God to help me learn about forgiveness. I came to see that forgiving someone doesn't mean I condone the wrong; it means I accept that it happened and let go of judgment. After all, Nothing, absolutely nothing, happens in God's world by mistake Until I could accept my sexaholism, I could not stay sober (*AA* 417).

I began to accept others without resentment and slowly became willing to make amends for the wrongs I did to them, regardless of what they had done to me. An unexpected result of this was that I began to accept myself in a more loving way.

*3*

When I first looked at Step Eight, I thought I already had my list of harms from Step Four, so I decided I should just go on to

Step Nine. The key words were, "*I thought . . . I decided.*" When I considered making my amends, I ran into a wall. I delayed and spent all my time thinking about the hardest amends and the ones I couldn't see any way to make because the people involved were anonymous or dead. The longer I waited, the bigger my imagined list became.

As time went by, I became more and more anxious about my lack of progress. I eventually talked with my sponsor about it. He told me to make a list of all the people I had harmed, not only those on my Fourth Step inventory but also those who had been indirectly affected by what I had done (their children, spouse, employer, etc.). I did what has been consistently important in my recovery—I followed directions.

The process of making a list was a critical one for me. It brought me back to reality. The other part of the Step—becoming willing—included praying, writing, and getting feedback from my sponsor.

Next, my sponsor asked me to prioritize the names from easiest to hardest. As I looked at the top of the list, I could actually imagine making amends to the easier ones. I found that I was already willing to make the first few. I now began to have hope and confidence that I really could "make amends to them all."

*4*

I told my sponsor I was ready to make one of my amends. He told me to write a draft of what I would say during the amends. When I showed him the draft, he helped me see that some of what I had planned to say might actually be harmful. As I rewrote drafts and shared them with my sponsor, I saw my tendency to rationalize, justify, and explain what I had done. He suggested I keep it short, admit my wrongs, and ask how I could make it right. These written "scripts" were a great reference for me later when I was nervous about making the amends.

*5*

Some time after completing Steps Eight and Nine, I realized that there were people I had harmed who were not on my earlier list. I would need to revisit Step Eight to maintain my recovery.

I also saw that I needed to broaden my understanding of what harm I might have caused. For example, I came to see that my acting-out partners had been harmed in more ways than I had originally thought. In our affairs, my partners and I had created a secret life. None of them felt free to tell their family members about our affair. So in taking advantage of my acting-out partners, I was disrupting the relationship between them and their families. I discovered that, like ripples in a pond when an object is thrown into the water, my affairs had effects that went far beyond my actions.

*6*

As I worked Step Eight I learned about the difference between *becoming* willing and *feeling* willing. When resentment or fear contributed to my feeling of unwillingness, I had to remember a program slogan my sponsor had taught me: "Take the action and the feelings will follow." Sometimes I found that the feeling of forgiveness toward others and myself came when I made amends. If I had not taken the action, I might never have felt it. *Sexaholics Anonymous* quotes one member's experience with this problem:

> Regardless of how I tried, I just could not bring myself to feel forgiving.
> . . . [But] I could admit I was powerless over it, do a Step One, Two, and Three on it, and give it up to God. Then I just asked for the willingness to take the action anyway, first in my heart. And it wasn't long before I could hear myself in my mind saying, 'Dad, I forgive you."
>
> The book points the lesson for me: "We take the action of forgiving, even when we don't feel forgiving" (*SA* 125).

Because I did not always feel forgiving toward others, it helped me when my sponsor told me that "forgiveness is giving up the right to get back at someone." Surrendering my right to get revenge was easier for me than trying to generate feelings of forgiveness.

*7*

While working Step Eight, I realized that if I could love people who had hurt me, perhaps I could be loved by those I had hurt. If I could forgive, then perhaps I could be forgiven. I used to think that forgiving someone meant letting them off the hook. But if I control the hook, then I decide when to let them off. That's far too much power in the hands of someone as powerless as I am. Today, I find more peace in believing that forgiveness is about realizing there is no hook.

*8*

My sponsor advised me I should postpone my amends to several of the people on my list. He said that even though I wanted to make amends to them, I might not be able to make direct amends without doing further harm. But I didn't realize that I should still do my Eighth Step work and prepare to make amends to these people.

A short time later I unexpectedly ran into a woman with whom I had had an affair. There had been a lot of publicity so she knew that I had lost my job over my acting out. We spoke and I told her of my SA program. I said that I knew I had hurt her and wanted to make amends to her, but I felt inadequate to the situation and apologized for not being more prepared. God seemed to take care of things. She accepted my amends and told me that reading the publicity about my consequences had a profound effect on her. She herself had undergone a religious conversion and had renewed her commitment to her marriage. She said that although it had been painful for her, she was now grateful for what she had been through and what she had found. She held no ill will toward me. We parted and have not seen each other again in the intervening years.

That event helped me realize that whether I thought I would be able to make direct amends or not, I should prepare to make all my amends. I can never know when God will decide to place one of these people in my day. I began to write my amends for *all* the people on my list. I cannot be completely willing to make amends until I am fully prepared to make them. For me that includes clarity about how I feel, what I believe, and what I have to say and do as amends. The other realization I had was that making amends is another part of my life that I don't control but only participate in. I must be willing and do what's in front of me, but God is the One who makes it happen.

*9*

I asked an SA member if he would hear my Eighth Step. He had four more years of sobriety than I. He agreed to hear it and suggested I write as long a list as possible along with some mention of the harm done. I did so.

We met an hour before an SA meeting in a side room. I went down the list one name at a time, pencil ready. In each case, the harm I had done was direct and obvious. The relationship was permanently altered, if not ruined. Those named included my wife, former wife, children, a cousin, an employee, a department store, and one woman I had treated unfairly. Some would be living amends and some would be direct amends. I remember being amazed and relieved at the end of our session. I had a list. While it would not be easy, I could make amends to them all. It was at this moment I knew that completing the Twelve Steps of SA would be possible for me.

*10*

By the time I arrived at Step Eight, I was pleased that I had already made a list of people I had harmed in my Fourth Step inventory. I re-examined that list and added a few more names.

In order to make amends to those on the list, I was instructed to write a letter to each, spelling out exactly what I had done to hurt each one, and what I would do to make amends. Some of the letters were to groups of people and some were anonymous since I didn't know their names. These letters were a spiritual exercise in becoming willing to forgive myself, willing to forgive those I hurt, and willing to make it right—that is, "willing to make amends to them all."

It was difficult for me to forgive the people to whom I was

getting ready to admit my wrongs. I had to remind myself continually of how pointless and hypocritical it would be to attempt amends to someone I would not forgive. When I was unwilling to forgive, I asked God to help me forgive them, as often as necessary, whether I wanted to or not. Repeatedly asking for His help eventually worked, as it always has when I have asked with sincerity.

The words of *Sexaholics Anonymous* on "Step Eight and One-Half" were a help in this process:

> Practicing forgiveness in our hearts as we think of these people, then aloud, perhaps even with our sponsor, we forgive every person on our list and keep on forgiving them every time the resentment returns. We may find it necessary to forgive and pray for them each time we think about them until we are free of the resentment. The willingness and the gift of love do come if we persist (125-126).

## *Step into Action*

### *Recommended Readings*

We suggest that members read and study the following before working the Step:

*Alcoholics Anonymous* (*AA*)
"Chapter 6" 76-84

*Sexaholics Anonymous* (*SA*)
Steps Eight and Nine 123-128

*Twelve Steps and Twelve Traditions* (*12&12*)
"Step Eight" 77-82

## *One Method for Working Step Eight*

Prayerfully, we prepare a list of the persons we have harmed. If making the list triggers an emotional or lustful reaction, we pray or pick up the phone and share what we are experiencing with another member. We remind ourselves that we are doing the right thing, undertaking a courageous endeavor.

It is useful to review what we mean by "harm." The *12&12* is helpful here:

> To define the word "harm" in a practical way, we might call it the result of instincts in collision, which cause physical, mental, emotional, or spiritual damage to people. If our tempers are consistently bad, we arouse anger in others. If we lie or cheat, we deprive others not only of their worldly goods, but of their emotional security and peace of mind. We really issue them an invitation to become contemptuous and vengeful. If our sex conduct is selfish, we may excite jealousy, misery, and a strong desire to retaliate in kind (*12&12* 80).

This description of harms we may have done continues in the text and also merits review.

> We start by praying and writing a list of names based on our Fourth Step inventory and on a review of our character defects. Alongside each name we jot down a few words to remind us of the harm we have done. The actual writing of the initial list can take less than an hour. Since the Step calls for a list of *all* the people we had harmed, we consider the family and friends of those involved. Have any of them been affected? Have our acts caused someone to neglect his or her spouse or children? Did our actions have indirect effects on the person's co-workers or customers? We prayerfully ask to

> be reminded of names we may have omitted. As additional individuals come to mind, we write down their names. The *12&12* tells us to make our list as thorough as possible, *without regard to the action we may take in Step Nine* (*12&12* 78-9).

With input from our sponsor, we often reorder our list. A common practice is to begin with the amends we are more willing to make and gradually move to those we are less willing to make. We often find that our willingness to make the more difficult amends increases as we work our way through the list. We do not necessarily need to make amends in this order, but many have found this method helpful.

We found it helps to prepare our amends as soon as we write the list. To this end, many of us write a "script" of what words we will say as amends to each person. As we write, we often find that additional healing words or indicated actions come to mind that would make our amends more complete. Whether the people on our list are alive or dead, whether their whereabouts are known or unknown, or whether or not we will be able to make direct amends to them, it is helpful to write a brief script and pray about what else needs to be done in each case. We continue to review our scripts and our plans with our sponsor.

These scripts are free of excuses for our behavior or comments about the wrongs others may have done. We identify our own wrongs and acknowledge our responsibility. Some find it helpful to follow the suggestion on page 100 of *Sexaholics Anonymous*:

> *The words, 'I was wrong,' which I was forever trying to extort from others, become, when I make them mine, the most wonderful words in the world. They bring peace to me! How can something that felt so bad turn into such a great good.*
>
> The key to recovery and spiritual growth is the righting of our wrongs. It dissolves our guilt, sets us free, and energizes us with joy and strength.

> *Righting our wrongs thus becomes the single most powerful tool for success in spiritual growth and recovery.* Why? (1) It gets the wrong out of the way so God can work in us. (2) Taking such repeated actions begins to loosen the hold over us of one defect at a time (*SA* 101).

Completing this work for everyone on our list helps us become willing to make amends. This work brings us healing. As we find forgiveness for others and as we experience the forgiveness of our Higher Power, we find we are more capable to forgive ourselves. One of the gifts of working Steps Eight and Nine is removal of the shame and guilt related to our harms.

Step Eight is a tool to be used for the rest of our lives. We are human. We will continue to harm others through the years, and we may be reminded, from time to time, of harms long forgotten. With perseverance and our Higher Power's help and guidance, we become willing to make amends. Then we are ready to move on to Step Nine.

## *Some Questions to Consider*

1. Am I willing to set aside one hour a week to write my initial list?
2. Have I made a start by writing down the names taken from my Fourth Step inventory? What is my start date?
3. Alongside each name have I jotted down a brief description of the harm I have done?
4. Are there amends you are afraid to make? How can your relationship with God help you?
5. Am I prayerfully asking God to be reminded of names I may have omitted?
6. Am I willing to make amends to all the people on my list?
7. Am I willing to pray for willingness to forgive people on my list for harms they may have done to me?
8. Have I put my name on this list? Why or why not?
9. Have I listed exercises, such as Program or other spiritual practices, that can help me to forgive myself for harms I have done to others and myself?
10. Am I willing to meet with my sponsor or another sober person to review my list in detail and the harms I caused before I take Step Nine? Why should I do this before I make any amends or edit the list? Will I make an accurate/complete and really exhaustive survey of my past life? Do I believe that it will lead to eventual freedom from bondage of self?

# *Step Nine*

*Made direct amends to such people wherever possible, except when to do so would injure them or others*

In making amends, we took action to bring honesty and healing to relationships we had damaged. We did everything in our power to correct our lies and the damage we had inflicted in the past. Accomplishing this while avoiding further harm required prayerful consideration and the counsel of others.

Although we might get a positive response when we made amends to those we had harmed, we did not make amends in order to obtain forgiveness or approval. We made amends because the process was necessary for our recovery. As a result of these somewhat difficult actions, we stayed sober, continued to grow and develop as human beings, and began to realize the promises of recovery. We took responsibility for our actions, expressed regret, corrected our behavior, and made restitution where appropriate. Without expectation, we often experienced healing in both ourselves and those we harmed.

While an apology can be part of an amends, apologies alone are generally insufficient. It may be true that we have been sorry throughout much of our lives, but such admissions generally have not led to necessary changes in our thinking and behavior. Sometimes, before recovery, we misused apologies to make excuses, to shift blame, or to avoid unpleasant consequences of our actions. Sometimes we brought up details of our past that reopened old wounds. In this way, we tried to lighten our burden at the expense of others, selfishly trying to shed our own guilt and remorse. This was not the purpose of Step Nine.

In approaching Step Nine, we let go of our expectations of other people's responses to our amends. Some of those on our list remembered our wrongdoing, while others had no recollection of incidents about which we had felt guilty for years. The people we had harmed often accepted and appreciated our amends. Sometimes they reciprocated in kind. On the rare occasion when we were rejected, we remembered that we were doing the right thing: we were clearing away our past wrongs to make room for spiritual growth. Other people's responses were their business. Our business was to do our part and leave the results to God.

We made direct amends *wherever possible,* in our present situation, with our present means. Whenever we could, we made amends in person, as this is most beneficial to us. However, when it was not possible to visit someone we telephoned or sent a letter. Trying to do the impossible, we learned, was not the solution. We did what we could, and we were willing and open to doing more if we had the ability in the future. Willingness was the key, and counsel with our sponsor and others would keep our character defects from causing further harm.

We had to be willing to accept the consequences of our actions, even if that meant loss of jobs, or financial, or legal difficulties. However, we had to avoid doing injury to those we had harmed and to others who might be affected by a revelation of our past misdeeds, such as our spouse or children.

> There can only be one consideration which should qualify our desire for a complete disclosure of the damage we have done. That will arise in the occasional situation where to make a full revelation would seriously harm the one to whom we are making amends. Or—quite as important—other people (*12&12* 86).

If there were people who were dependent upon us, they had to be considered. But this couldn't be used as an excuse to avoid making things right. There were many ways to cause further injury by our amends, and we were often blind to them. We discussed these matters with our sponsor, with other sober members, and, where appropriate, with those who might be affected. We had faith that, whatever happened, God would take care of us all.

When we weren't sure what to do in a particular situation, we prayed for guidance, talked about it with our sponsor and others, and waited—sometimes for uncomfortably long periods. The proper course of action became clear in God's time, not in ours. We eventually saw how we could make things right without causing further harm. We often had to trust the wisdom of other sober members. We had to be willing to do the right thing when we knew what it was. Waiting out of fear never improved the situation. We might have feared the consequences, or worried about not getting it right, or been afraid of one of the many other things that could go wrong when we ran the show. By avoiding our amends out of selfish concern, we risked depriving ourselves of some of the deepest spiritual joy the program has to offer. So we confronted our fear, accepted responsibility for our behavior, and resolved to make the best amends we could.

For direct amends we sought to make reparations to those we had harmed, financially or otherwise. In some situations, we could only acknowledge our responsibility and our regret, and change our behavior.

> There's no feeling in all the world like having mended a long-standing wrong. It is better than the relief that comes from finally pulling a thorn from a festering finger., more like pulling a thorn from our festering soul. Soul surgery... We courageously come face to face, not only with that other person we've avoided, but with ourselves---the real monster we've been fleeing all our lives. Then, when we've done it, there's a marvelous sense of accomplishment, release, and great joy. Why did we ever wait so long? (*SA* 127)

When we could not contact people, or if by so doing we risked harming them or others, we made indirect amends. These usually consisted of taking positive action related to the harm we had done, while not directly involving the one we had harmed.

> Few things can so damage the possibility of healing in the family as a premature confession to spouse or family where sacred bonds and trust have been violated. Unwittingly, such confessions can be attempts on our part to dump our guilt,

get back into good graces, or make just another show of willpower (*SA* 128-129).

In all cases, we were able to make living amends. As *Twelve Steps and Twelve Traditions* tells us, "we consider how, with our newfound knowledge of ourselves, we may develop the best possible relations with every human being we know" (77).

Writing out an amend and then reading it to our sponsor as a review (and as if they were the person to whom we were making amends) is a great way to ensure accuracy.

Working Step Nine, we saw obstacles dissolve and seemingly impossible situations resolve in unexpected ways. By making amends, we gained the courage of faith.

## *Members of SA Share*

### *1*

In approaching Step Nine, I felt a sense of dread. The process included some very difficult door-knocking experiences. Particularly painful and humbling were my amends to my spouse, children, and other family members. After getting through the tough ones, I found myself filled with gratitude, relief, and contentment. Much to my surprise, I found this Step to be an opportunity to know God's grace more fully. It is an awesome undertaking to right our own wrongs, completely leaving aside the wrongs done to us. There is nothing like being able to look at my Eighth Step list, with amends made to all, and to know that I have done everything within my power to fix what I have broken. The Ninth Step experience remains one of the most important and fulfilling chapters of my life.

### *2*

I didn't know how to make amends to my aborted child and the victims of my exhibitionism, but I knew I must. Just praying for them was not enough. I needed to do something so that these prayers would be real. I prayed for guidance and sought direction from my sponsor. I saw that it would be insane to try to make amends without help as I might do further harm.

Here are the amends I made and continue to make:

- I wrote letters to my aborted child and to each of my victims. I admitted my wrongs and prayed that each would be filled with God's love and peace. I read my letter to my child at his grave. I was told not to send the letters to the other victims but to give them to God.
- When the memories of my victims come back, I pray to be able to see them as God sees them and to love them as God loves them.
- I began the practice of donating blood.
- I make anonymous donations to a sexual assault treatment center.
- I contribute to the financial support of a child in another country.

Somehow in this process I experienced forgiveness. I became able to forgive myself. My sponsor taught me that there is always some way to make a tangible amends. I have learned much about myself in the process. My spirit grows when I actually do something to make amends. Thank God for physical, tangible action!

*3*

My Fourth Step inventory revealed in great detail the physical, emotional, and spiritual harm I had done to my wife. I had battered her self-esteem and threatened her security. I had lied. I had broken promises.

In my direct amends, I told her the truth about who I was and what I had done (in a way that avoided doing further harm). I righted the wrong of lying by telling the truth. I acknowledged the ways I had harmed her. I asked if she had anything to add, and I listened to her response. As living amends, I began treating her in a more loving manner. Amending something is about righting a wrong, improving something. So my behavior toward her had to change, and slowly it has.

*4*

For years I blamed my father for my problems and told anyone who would listen how badly he had abused me. Even though he died many years before my recovery began, it remained a difficult relationship for me. I struggled to become willing to make amends to him. After a lot of prayer, journaling, and talking with my sponsor, I was blessed with forgiveness for him and willingness to amend the relationship. For Step Nine, I wrote a letter that I shared with him at his grave and committed to these ongoing living amends.

I resolved to tell only good stories about him to my children and others. Even in recovery situations I have been able to share my experience in this relationship without putting my father in a bad light. This was a major change in my behavior. I resolved not to blame him for my problems anymore. When the temptation arose, I reminded myself that I had been granted forgiveness and surrendered the negative thoughts. Before long these thoughts ceased. I resolved to have relationships with my children that I believe my father would have liked to have had with me. I resolved to have relationships with my siblings and my mother that I believe my father would have wanted me to have.

There used to be darkness around my memory of my father. Now, there are positive stories and acts of kindness.

*5*

I am a member of an organization that is polarized. For years, I participated in isolating from and gossiping about the majority, becoming more interested in vilification than reconciliation. I had treated others with disrespect, and I put this behavior on my Eighth Step list.

I could not see how to make amends, but after prayer and consultation God showed me a way. With the approval of my sponsor, at an annual retreat attended by members of both the minority and the majority, I asked to speak. I apologized to the members of the majority who were there. Although they were not necessarily individuals that I had issues with or had spoken against, they stood in proxy for those I had abused. They gratefully received and accepted my amends; I was gratefully freed.

*6*

My Eighth Step list included those people I had used to feed my addiction. Whether in the media or in person, I had contributed to the humiliation, degradation, and dehumanization of many children of God. Direct amends were impractical.

My sponsor approved the following actions: I found an organization far away that works with prostitutes, helping them to make changes and find a more productive and self-affirming direction. I send regular, anonymous donations to this organization. Daily, as well as whenever they come to mind, I pray for God to help those who are abused in the sex industry. I volunteer at a homeless shelter. Each year I give some money to another SA member to distribute to needy people at his discretion. I ask not to be told where the money goes. I pray to be guided to whatever else I can do to set things right. It will take the rest of my life, but today I feel better knowing that I am a positive influence in the world and that I'm not using or abusing people anymore.

*7*

I couldn't forgive myself. The shameful feelings from the things I had done were still overwhelming. My memories still haunted me. My perceptions of myself were still negative—even after fifteen years of sobriety.

I cried. I was humbled. I finally realized that I needed much more help than I had requested. Under the guidance of God and the sponsorship of a long-term sober member (who had worked the Steps with a sponsor), I worked the Steps again—this time from the perspective that I knew nothing. I was taught that I needed to work *all* the Steps thoroughly, with rigorous honesty, in order to experience the promise of recovery. I believed that God forgave me, but I could not experience that forgiveness until I took action. Acceptance of God's forgiveness began with Step Four and was fully realized with Step Nine. The actions I took to make amends helped me to believe that I had changed. I was no longer a person who did perverted things.

*8*

I had a long list of friends and family members I had harmed by disappearing, being unreliable, and generally putting my addiction before my relationships with them. As I started into Step Nine, I was frightened and had to surrender that fear to my Higher Power. But as I worked my way through my list, I saw a pattern emerge. God was using the amends process to work on one of my primary character defects: my inability to receive love.

I was blown away, amends after amends, by how my friends all said a variation of the same thing: I love you. Of course I forgive you. You were such an important part of my life, and I missed you when you spiraled into your addiction. But now, you're back, but as a new version of your old self. I can see how all the hard work you're doing is paying off. And I'm glad to have you back, better than ever.

One amends at a time, God is helping me see that I am worthy of their love, and teaching me how to accept it.

*9*

I approached my Ninth Step a lot like I did my Fourth. Avoidance! So much emotional wreckage was packed away that I was terrified to stir it up and actually see it. Especially the hurts I had caused. When I got around to acting, actually doing Step work, I was "amazed before I was half way through" (*AA* 83).

I am learning to work the Steps as they are suggested, so I picked a few "easy" amends to do first. I was overwhelmed with the loving responses. One was my ex-wife's uncle. I still call him Uncle Merle, but hadn't talked to him during my past decade of active addiction. A favorite uncle, he held deep affection for my ex-wife and me. During the 21 years of our marriage he was always a positive force.

For amends, we met at the dining place of his retirement home. Right away, I was amazed at how happy he was to spend time together. Almost as if my amends were secondary to simply catching up. I still get a little misty-eyed when remembering. Some of the Twelve Step Promises really came true that day. I almost couldn't handle getting the good shaming I felt I deserved.

He was overjoyed to hear of my addiction recovery process,

and got a little misty-eyed himself. He is perhaps the best listener, conversationalist, and mentor that I've known. He always "got me," and helped me get myself, and the same thing happened that day as we talked. He shared the past decade of his own life that I had missed. I felt a moment of grief, knowing I had traded this connection for the misconnection of my lust addiction.

Then a moment of sanity hit me in what came next. Decades earlier, his son had been the victim of a church sexual abuse cover-up, resulting in the son's suicide. My profession involved me in these kinds of matters, so I had been a confidant and support to Uncle Merle and his family for many years. As usual he shared more of his journey about this.

He used the term "sexual predator." What came crashing in to my now sober brain was that I realized for the first time that I was also a sexual predator. (I've had to practice actually saying that out loud, and can now share it in SA meetings.) I could finally see myself. I felt like my whole brain was getting re-arranged. I had crossed the same professional sexual boundaries that had destroyed his son. I was in a daze—the shock of truth. How could it be, all during those years of listening and caring for my uncle's family tragedy, I was grooming and abusing clients? I was creating tragedies, and didn't see the very obvious parallels. How could I not know! I saw vividly the "cunning, baffling and powerful" distortion of lust. The words "sexual predator" registered for the first time and sank in with the impact of knowing my uncle's inner torture all those years.

I may never speak to those clients or their husbands or their families. I may never tell my uncle these details. But I am very grateful to have restored my relationship with Uncle Merle as a living amends, and am so grateful to be restored to some measure of mental sanity.

As I finished my amends with my dear uncle, marveling at the blessings God had just provided, half a dozen of my ex-wife's family members walked into the room. They rushed over with smiles and hugs. (My sponsor says he doesn't believe in coincidences—he believes in God-incidences.) How could I be so forgiven?

## *Recommended Readings*

We suggest that members read and study the following before working the Step:

*Alcoholics Anonymous* (*AA*)
Chapter Six 76 - 84

*Sexaholics Anonymous* (*SA*)
Step Nine 126 - 128

*Twelve Steps and Twelve Traditions* (*12&12*)
Step Nine 83-87

## *One Method for Working Step Nine*

We hurt others out of self-will and self-centered fear. Working Step Nine *on our own* will usually perpetuate this problem. When making amends to someone we have harmed, we are careful to avoid causing further harm. *Before* contacting the person, we discuss with our sponsor the specific wrong and *exactly* how we will make the amends. Another member can often see the danger in our plan when we cannot. They can catch the remaining character defects at work in our planned amends, when we are blind to them. Decades of experience in this program are available to us if we just ask.

When we owe amends to people who have harmed us we may feel awkward or afraid. These amends can be difficult, yet they offer tremendous opportunities for growth. When we practice acceptance of others and of our mistakes, the humility we learn is the door to freedom. *Alcoholics Anonymous* counsels us,

> It is harder to go to an enemy than to a friend, but we find it much more beneficial to us. We go to him in a helpful and forgiving spirit, confessing our former ill feeling and expressing our regret. Under no condition do we criticize such a person. Simply we tell him that we will never get over [lusting] until we have done our utmost to straighten out the past (77).

We are careful to make our amends to the appropriate person. If we gossiped about someone, we make amends to the person *to* whom we gossiped, not the person *about* whom we gossiped (unless our words caused direct harm). If we have harbored a hostile attitude toward someone but didn't do any direct harm, we *don't* tell the person directly of our ill will. We confess our ill will to our sponsor and ask for guidance.

In making amends for illegal actions we pray for the willingness to accept the consequences. We have to be willing to go to any length for our recovery. It is a matter of survival. We should neither avoid responsibility nor thoughtlessly make ourselves or others vulnerable. Again, discussion with our sponsor and, where appropriate, with those who might be affected by our amends is essential.

Direct amends are best made face-to-face. When that is not possible, we use the telephone or send a carefully worded letter that has been reviewed by our sponsor. For those who have died, we can visit cemeteries and make graveside amends.

When we are ready to make direct amends, we think about where to meet for the amends. We consider meeting in a quiet, neutral place, taking into account the other person's comfort. If we are concerned about being alone with this person, we can choose a public place. In some situations, it makes sense to have another member nearby. For example, one member, out of consideration for her husband's concern, decided it would be unwise for her to meet alone with some of the people to whom she owed amends.

We prepare by reviewing the scripts we prepared in Step Eight and praying before the meeting. We ask that we will "be sensible, tactful, considerate and humble without being servile or scraping" (*AA* 83). It is important to keep our amends brief to guard against rationalization, justification, defensiveness, or blame. Unlike our Fourth Step, in Step Nine we address our harmful behavior, not the inner workings of our disease. One common formula for an amends is "I was wrong to ______; I ask your forgiveness." If our amends include reparation, for example in money, service, or replacement of damaged belongings, we negotiate that. "Arranging the best deal we can we let these people know we are sorry" (*AA* 78). Often our amends spark a conversation with the other person, but if not, when we are finished we may ask if they have anything they would like to add. We may ask the person what we can do to make things right. We are prepared to listen to what the other person has to say, but it could be unwise to agree to any unforeseen restitution without first discussing it with our sponsor.

After completing a direct amends, we often contact another member and tell them what we have done, how it went, and how we feel. This gives us the opportunity to remember what we are trying to accomplish and remind ourselves that we are doing the right thing. Especially after difficult conversations, it helps to reflect on what might be bothering us and to surrender our fears with another.

In some cases, we make indirect amends. This category includes people we cannot find, people we harmed who are anonymous, people we cannot contact because they or someone else would be injured by that action, and people who have died.

There are many ways to make indirect amends. For example, we can do community service for, and/or make anonymous donations to, organizations that help people harmed in ways similar to the harm we have done; or we can perform some service anonymously in an area of our community where we used to act out. It is important here that our amends be appropriate to the damage we caused. A one-time contribution might not be sufficient for years of abuse. We ask our Higher Power, our sponsor, and others for help in deciding how to make indirect amends appropriate to the person and the injury.

An essential part of any amends is changing our behavior, what we call "living amends." We go forward, living a sober life and behaving well toward those who are in our life. We begin practicing a positive sobriety, taking the actions of love to improve our relations with others. We were learning how to give; and the measure we gave was a measure we got back (*SA* 205). We refrain from the behaviors that caused harm in the past. We take positive actions that we had neglected to take, recognizing that if we had done so before we might not have needed to make amends.

As we begin to repair the damage we have done, we see the value of correcting our mistakes as soon as we are able. To that end, even while we continue to work Step Nine we move on and begin the process of Step Ten.

If we are painstaking about this phase of our development, we will be amazed before we are half way through. We are going to know a new freedom and a new happiness (*AA* 83).

## *Some Questions to Consider*

1. Am I willing to review my planned amends with my sponsor before approaching the persons I owe amends to?
2. Have I reviewed in detail with my sponsor my motives for making each individual amends?
3. Am I willing to accept the outcome of the amends, whatever it may be?
4. Are there amends I need to make but am postponing out of fear? What steps can I take toward making them?
5. Have I planned for other ways to make amends whenever direct amends are not possible?
6. How will I make amends to those who have died?
7. Are there amends to make to myself? How can I make them?
8. Which amends can best be done by changes in my behavior? What changes?
9. In *Alcoholics Anonymous* there is a list of Ninth Step "Promises" on pages 83-4. Are any of these promises being fulfilled in my life today?

# *Step Ten*

### *Continued to take personal inventory and when we were wrong promptly admitted it.*

In our addiction, we routinely tried to convince ourselves we were right even when we knew we were wrong. This was one of the first unsettling truths about ourselves we had to face when we came into the Fellowship. Fortunately for most of us, however, it was also one of the first truths about ourselves we became willing to change. Encouraged by the example of others in SA, we began the sometimes painful journey of growing our capacity to be honest with ourselves, others and God. If we were to stay sober and grow in recovery, it became clear we would have to learn to make honesty a way of life.

Each Step, beginning with our admittance in Step One that we were sexaholics and could not manage our own lives, required a degree of honesty. In Step Two we took an honest look at the spiritual beliefs, or lack thereof, that enabled us to persist in destructive thinking and behavior.

In Step Three we find our true connection or lose our self! We discovered that the root of our problem is conscious separation from the Source of our lives; the solution is conscious union with that Source. Steps Four through Nine introduced us to critical recovery practices based on rigorous honesty, including self-inventory, telling on ourselves, and making amends for our wrongs. Step Ten required that we practice these new skills on an ongoing basis, thereby incorporating them into our daily lives.

We noticed from the beginning that Step Ten required us to admit instances *when,* not *if,* we were wrong. This told us that even as we grew in recovery, we would continue to make mistakes. Among other benefits, Step Ten freed us of the notion that we could or should be perfect.

As we accepted that we would be wrong from time to time, we recognized the wisdom of the suggestion in *Alcoholics Anonymous* that "we continue to take personal inventory and continue to set right any new mistakes as we go along." In particular, we continue "to watch for selfishness, dishonesty, resentment, and fear" (84). In earlier Steps we used the inventory process to find our errors in thinking and behavior. In Step Ten, ongoing personal inventory and quick amends kept the mistakes of the present from becoming the wreckage of the past.

We learned in Step Four that before we could see our mistakes clearly we had to surrender resentments against those who had wronged us.

> We realized that the people who wronged us were perhaps spiritually sick. Though we did not like their symptoms and the way these disturbed us, they, like ourselves, were sick too. We asked God to help us show them the same tolerance, pity, and patience that we would cheerfully grant a sick friend (*AA* 66).

Step Ten challenged us to continue this process on a daily and sometimes hourly basis. It is a spiritual axiom that every time we are disturbed, no matter what the cause, there is something wrong *with us* (*12 & 12* 90). First, we accepted that each time we were disturbed by the words or actions of another person, this disturbance told us there was something in ourselves that we needed to change. We learned to avoid reacting to or blaming others. We began to develop self-restraint (*12&12* 91, meaning that we sought serenity before taking actions— reflecting and connecting, so that we could respond rationally rather than reacting as a slave to our feelings. Similarly, we tempered our responses to positive news and events, for in our self-centered way we had also done harm to ourselves and others by boasting of our perceived good fortune, or by losing ourselves in euphoria. Each time we had wronged others by our words or actions, we practiced Step Ten by promptly admitting our error.

When troubled, we gained valuable perspective by pausing, praying for clarity, and asking to be relieved of pride, fear, and self-centeredness. We talked to another sober member before responding to difficult situations. This allowed us the time and distance we needed to detach from events. When we were hasty, we risked causing more harm. If we were unable to make a decision, we continued to pray and surrender to God. After consultation with others, we sometimes found that no further action was necessary.

At other times we saw that we needed to admit our wrong. It was progress for us to honestly recognize and admit to ourselves each time we had made a mistake. However, recognizing and admitting it to ourselves was usually not enough. For many of us, admitting we were wrong was unfamiliar. Fear told us that if we were wrong we were not worthwhile. Being wrong felt life-threatening. We had spent lots of time and energy proving to others that we were right. If we couldn't do that, the next best thing was to prove that others were wrong. Practicing Step Ten therefore became our primary tool for becoming rightly related to ourselves, others and God. When appropriate, we admitted our wrong to the other person and took the action necessary to make things right. Taking action promptly is key in working Step 10.

A simple admission of our error had a profound positive effect on us and on those close to us. We experienced a new sense of freedom and felt the burden of guilt lift as we forgave ourselves. As we practiced self-restraint we began to see situations where we could be helpful. Detachment allowed us to see that other people were also imperfect and gave us compassion for their struggles. We saw that becoming angry or upset over human shortcomings, whether our own or others', was a waste of time and energy (*12&12* 92). We were learning from our mistakes, and as we saw that being wrong could be a gift to our humility and sometimes even a useful human characteristic, we became more tolerant of others and ourselves.

> Forgiving another is a divine an act as we humans can ever aspire to. It's as hard or harder to say "I forgive you" as it is to admit wrong. But we can and must forgive.
>
> The highest reach of the soul is outward toward another in this motion of reconciliation. Step 10 is the great maker of true spiritual union (*SA* 130).

As we continued to admit and correct our wrongs in the present, our past was no longer filled with shame and guilt. We became more open to the spiritual life. Continuing to take personal inventory was a life-sustaining and life-enhancing process, necessary for growing closer to our Higher Power. This discipline of honest self-reflection was our path to happiness and serenity. These were the fruits of our efforts and of our improving spiritual condition.

> Making amends seems to be what gives me the most practice in changing my defects of character. It makes me think twice before opening my big mouth, knowing how painful the prospect of making amends will be (*SA* 131).

## *Members of SA Share*

### *1*

For my daily Tenth Step inventory I journal each morning while the water is heating for my coffee. The journal is in the form of a personal letter to God on the following topics: my feelings, how I'm doing, and whatever resentments and fears I am harboring. I simply pour out the truth on these matters. I get right to the point and just let it flow. It can be as little as one page or as many as four. This is what I bring to God in my quiet time before work—either during my morning commute or lying on a mat on the floor of my office. Later, I read it to my sponsor and listen to his perspective on it. This little spiritual exercise has allowed me to be accountable for my feelings and actions. I also read this journal entry to other SA members I talk with that day. It helps me to remember that I am in recovery and trying to go through the day in that spirit.

Once a month, I reread what I have written in my journal since the previous month. This allows me to see patterns developing where I may need to take action. There have been times when I thought I was doing well, but my journal showed me that I was taking daily lust hits in the commuter train, shuttle bus, and cafeteria at work. I had thought I was only allowing an occasional glance or thought, but my journal showed me the true extent of my laxity. This realization scared me enough to work and pray to shore up these weak places in my program. This is my method of continuing personal inventory. It has been very good for me because it teaches me to be honest with myself, with God, and with other people.

*2*

In working Step Ten, I put Steps Four through Nine into action on a daily and sometimes hourly basis. I often do my inventory in my head. Many times each day I observe my emotional state. When I feel myself begin to look for something wrong, I look for a person, principle, or institution associated with what I am feeling. After I look for the cause and what part of myself is threatened, usually my mistake becomes clear. I identify the associated fear, ask myself why I have it, look for how self-reliance has failed me, and consider how trusting and relying upon God might help. I ask God to remove the fear and direct my attention toward what He would have me be. I share with someone else, ask God to remove my short-comings, and make amends if necessary. When I get stumped somewhere in this process, a phone call to my sponsor helps me sort it out. With practice I have made progress. Sometimes I only have to feel bad for a few minutes before I can admit that I was wrong about something.

*3*

Today my daily review shows that I am holding on to a resentment that seems justified. Of course, as the program teaches me, holding onto a resentment is like drinking poison and hoping the other person dies. The good news is that, because of my new habit of personal inventory, I get to see my resentment and surrender it before it causes problems in my life. Then its power is gone. The program does not promise that my challenges will disappear—it promises me freedom to deal constructively with life's challenges. If I do the work, the problems will not dominate me anymore.

*4*

In addition to the spot-check inventory and the daily inventory, the AA *12 & 12* suggests a periodic, in-depth review with my sponsor. Therefore, on the occasion of my sobriety anniversary, I conduct a written evaluation of the state of my addiction and recovery and share it with other members and my sponsor. One method I have used is to write five headings on a piece of paper: New, Gone, Improving, Unchanged, and Worse. Under these headings I list qualities and attributes that describe my condition and behavior over the previous twelve months. Another method I have tried is to write descriptive paragraphs about what has gone on in my recovery and other areas of my life over the past year. Sharing this with my sponsor usually encourages me and shows me where I need to focus. With my sponsor's help I draw up an action plan to address areas that need attention.

Past action plans have included a wide variety of activities that, in one way or another, have strengthened my recovery. Actions I have taken include sending submissions to *Essay*, praying during my commute to work, exercising on a regular basis, reading for fun, and installing internet monitoring software on my home and work computers. When I stick to my action plan, my life improves.

*5*

The main thing I have learned about working Step Ten is to do it again and again. I can work a Tenth Step that takes minutes or hours, and I can work a Tenth Step that takes days or weeks. The objective is that I continue to work and grow to be more honest, considerate, unselfish, and loving. When I make mistakes along the way, I own up to them and make them right as soon as I can.

When I need to make amends I try to avoid saying, "I'm sorry." I feel as though I spent my whole life saying that, and it really describes what I was more than how I felt. Today, I say, "I was wrong about ____" or "I regret ____." I try to be specific about what I regret such as, "interrupting you" or "speaking to you harshly" or "being insensitive to your perspective" or "being aggressive."

Working the Steps is the solution to my problem. It is this process that replaces lust with "a happy and joyous freedom we could otherwise never know" (*SA* 202) and allows me "to be of maximum service to God and the people about [me]" (*AA* 77).

*6*

I always had a hard time admitting that I had made a mistake. When I was wrong I judged myself harshly and became afraid. The voices in my head told me I was bad, would be alone, and would be humiliated or punished, or maybe even dead, if anyone found out. This was especially true in my marriage and in my relationship with God. Those closest to me and most likely to forgive me were the ones I feared the most. When I was wrong, I was afraid and tongue-tied.

One night at a meeting I heard an answer to my dilemma. One member said that he had learned an all-purpose apology, "I'm sorry; I was wrong; please forgive me." Just eight simple words—easy to memorize and perfect for me. I began to use it with my spouse. It was sincere, honest, and short. I didn't have to think of what to say. I experienced tremendous relief by admitting my mistake. Gradually I have learned to be more specific when admitting my wrongs, but many times I still find it helpful to revert to those eight simple words.

*7*

When I'm too close to an uncomfortable situation and unable to see clearly where I am wrong, I may be unable to conduct a spot-check inventory. I have been taught a simple alternative. When I have erred but feel overwhelmed, I practice self-restraint and simply pray, "Thy will (not mine) be done" (*AA* 85).

Sometimes, however, I can't even get that far. If I am unjustly treated, I resist admitting any wrong because, quite frankly, I feel I shouldn't have to. This is where my Tenth Step reading hits me like a brick:

> It is a spiritual axiom that every time we are disturbed, no matter what the cause, there is something wrong *with us*. If somebody hurts us and we are sore, we are in the wrong also. But are there no exceptions to this rule? What about "justifiable" anger? If somebody cheats us, aren't we entitled to be mad? Can't we be properly angry with self-righteous folk? For us of [SA]

> these are dangerous exceptions. We have found that justified anger ought to be left to those better qualified to handle it (*12&12* 90).

Ouch! I am not qualified to handle anger? I get angry just by reading that! However, my personal history forces me to acknowledge that it is true. My life is a demonstration of my inability to handle anger. Anger is, as the *12&12* goes on to say, "that occasional luxury of more balanced people . . ." (90). This gets straight to the heart of the matter and I have come to accept this as true for me. So when I get angry these days, regardless of how legitimate that response may be, I let it go into God's care in humble recognition that I am part of the crowd that is completely and utterly unqualified to handle anger. This clears the way to admit where I am wrong.

It may be that I need to set a boundary or give myself some time or space, or that I am allowing someone else to take advantage of me. But I won't be able to see how to take care of myself as long as I am angry and focused on someone else's mistake.

*8*

Practicing the Tenth Step is a new way of living. For me it includes a morning routine. After prayer and admission of powerlessness to my Higher Power, I write down any resentments, fears, worries, lust hits, wrongs, and gratitudes. I then write down names of people I want to lift up to my Higher Power's care. I continue to practice the Tenth Step even though I am formally working on another Step.

*9*

The other day after a meeting, I pointed out to a member that he was shaming another member. He paused, and then asserted that I was now shaming him in front of others. I laughed and agreed, "You spot it; you got it." I realized that I did have it; I was shaming this fellow member. The right thing to do was to admit I was wrong right away and right there, admit my character defect and make amends.

## *Step into Action*

### *Recommended Readings*

We suggest that members read and study the following before working the Step:

*Alcoholics Anonymous* (*AA*)
"Chapter 6" 84-85

*Sexaholics Anonymous* (*SA*)
"Step Ten" 129-134

*Twelve Steps and Twelve Traditions* (*12&12*)
"Step Ten" 88-95

## *One Method of Working Step Ten*

Ours is a program of action, and the Tenth Step is no exception. The *12&12* outlines three types of personal inventory: the spot-check inventory, the daily inventory, and the periodic, in-depth review with a sponsor (89).

First, let us consider the spot-check inventory. Whenever we realize we are disturbed, we pause. The disturbance can manifest itself as anger, fear, excitement, a desire to be dishonest, the temptation to lust, or some other strong emotion. "Our first objective will be the development of self-restraint" (*12&12* 91).

We see that the term self-restraint is not implying that we can, by power of will and determination, ever control our lusting or force away our own character defects. That is God's job. What we can do is develop a healthier response to strong feelings and emotions. In our addiction, we could only ever react to strong feelings. The Steps provide a better answer. If through working Step Ten our "automatic response" becomes to inventory why we are feeling what we're feeling and then act on what we discover—either through surrender of an offending character defect to God, or making amends to right a wrong and heal a relationship—then, instead of simply reacting, we become more able to "do the next right thing!" We will be able to act on *His* will rather than our own. Emotional sobriety and serenity become possible. We are not developing any new power over our defects; we are simply learning how to stay connected with our Higher Power, and He becomes victorious over those defects.

Instead of reacting we practice making an honest analysis of what is going on. We ask ourselves questions such as these:

- What am I feeling?
- What mistake have I made or am I about to make?
- How is my thinking in error?
- What am I afraid of?
- What defect of character is motivating me?

We pray for guidance and the willingness to see our mistake and to forgive anyone who may be involved, including ourselves. We may need to take time out or make a phone call to see the situation clearly. Then we admit where we are wrong.

In short we *stop, look,* and *listen.* We *stop* what we are doing or saying. We *look* inside to see what is really going on with us. What are we doing, and why are we doing it? We *listen* for guidance from our Higher Power, from our sponsor, or from another sober member. We admit our fault to the extent that we are aware of it. We admit it to ourselves and to whomever necessary. By identifying the motivating character defect, we can continue to practice the opposite of that defect.

We do this promptly because the sooner we can admit our mistake, the sooner we are relieved and the less harm we will do. But we take the time we need. It is better to do it well than to be hasty and risk doing harm. Promptly means on time; it may mean on God's time, not ours. Sometimes we are unable to understand a situation in the heat of the moment. Reflection will make it clear if we are willing. We take care of it as soon as we can. If we struggle with the admission of wrong, we pray and continue our Step work.

Next, we establish a pattern of daily review. Many of us have found a daily written summary of the highs and lows of our thinking and behavior to be very helpful. We take note and express gratitude for things we have done well and for when we have been of service to others. We also take this opportunity to identify what we can do better and where we were thinking primarily of ourselves. We are able to share things that need to be shared and to make or plan amends when necessary. In this way we avoid taking today's problems into tomorrow.

For our daily review we have to establish a routine that works for us. The format may change over time. Daily review helps us identify recurring patterns of self-centered and self-defeating thoughts and actions. Identifying these helps us become willing to have them removed and motivates us to do our part to practice alternative behaviors. If we are to continue in recovery, we must change the thinking and behaviors that earned us a place in SA. We are careful not to use this as an exercise in self-judgment or self-hatred. Instead, we see our missteps as ongoing evidence of our powerlessness and our need for God, which can refresh and reinforce our Step One experience.

We may do this review as a part of our morning routine, on lunch break, during our commute, or before we retire at night. The important thing is that we do it and try to do it daily. As this becomes habit, we find we grow in self-restraint and tolerance of others.

We recognize the good along with the bad, so we get a complete picture of the day. We avoid losing ourselves in the negative, "for that would diminish our usefulness to others" (*AA* 86). For our daily inventory of credits, we look for what we have done well: constructive behaviors, good motives, healthy thoughts, kind actions, and even where we have tried but failed. We notice what principles we practiced that day and are grateful for times when God helped us to even small victories.

We find it useful, especially at first, to share our daily review with our sponsor or another sober member. Another person's perspective helps us see how we can improve and also see our progress.

A third type of inventory is a more in-depth inventory with our sponsor. For many of us this consists of repeating Steps Four and Five on a yearly basis. We have found that an annual review is well worth the time spent. Whatever we may have forgotten to include in our first Steps Four and Five will eventually be included in these inventories. This process helps us see our shortcomings and our progress. Through repeated inventories we watch some of our character defects nearly disappear while others seem to persist. We celebrate the former and continue to work on the latter.

> It is possible that, once relieved of the compulsion to act out our habit, we may feel cured and start coasting along with our tank on EMPTY. But the same personality defects that energized our addiction are still with us and, unattended, will take their toll again, sooner or later. Why are they still with us? Because they are us. Progressive victory over these defects, not their eradication is the power of God at work in us. It is a program of living. (*SA* 131).

Through the Steps, we have righted our wrongs to the best of our ability, and we continue to right them on a daily and hourly basis. Less impeded by our shortcomings and no longer hiding or fighting, we find ourselves more and more open to the Spiritual Life. Step Ten paves the way for us to pursue our relationship with God in Step Eleven.

## *Some Questions to Consider*

1. Am I willing to acquire "the habit of accurate self-appraisal" (*12&12* 89)? How can I acquire it?
2. What helps me to realize when I need to do a spot check inventory?
3. When is a good time during my day to do a daily inventory?
4. When was the last time I did an in-depth review with my sponsor? When is the next scheduled time?
5. Have I "ceased fighting anything or anyone" (*AA* 84)? With whom or what am I still fighting?
6. How does identifying and admitting my wrongs help me to "grow in understanding and effectiveness" (*AA* 84)?
7. Has my lust problem been removed? Am I "neither cocky nor afraid" when tempted to lust?

   (*AA* 84 – 85) What actions have I taken for these promises to come true?
8. What does it mean to me to "carry the vision of God's will into all of our activities" (*AA* 85)?
9. How does Step Ten help to maintain my spiritual condition?
10. Why is it important to promptly admit when I am wrong?

# *Step Eleven*

*Sought through prayer and meditation to improve our conscious contact with God as we understood Him, praying only for knowledge of His will for us and the power to carry that out.*

When our problems with life overwhelmed us, we sought relief in our addiction. For a while, lust appeared to be the answer. When we came to SA, we saw that lust was really the problem. We learned that the solution was coming to believe in a Power greater than ourselves.

Working the first ten Steps and attempting to practice right living in all our relationships, we grew nearer to the Power that guided our sobriety and our Step work. In Step Eleven, we focused on the practices we could take to further open ourselves to that Power—prayer and meditation.

> Just as surely as air is the breath of life for our bodies, prayer becomes the breath of life for our spirits. It is the means by which we make our Connection. Just as talking to another in the fellowship of forgiveness is the medium of life between people, so prayer as the expression of our inner being is the means by which we have fellowship with God. This is why we must learn to walk in the light. (*SA* 137).

Step Eleven can be described as a conversation with our Higher Power. As in any conversation we spend part of the time talking and part of the time listening. Prayer has been likened to talking and meditation to listening.

Before recovery, our prayers had been sporadic. Often we pleaded and bargained, "God, get me out of this and I will never do it again." Other times we prayed for God to do our bidding. Even when we professed good intentions, we were often asking for the power to accomplish our own will. That didn't work very well. If we got what we wanted, it still did not make us happy.

In early recovery many of us prayed and meditated only because the program literature or our sponsor suggested it. Soon we realized that we were getting practical results—prayer was helping us to stay physically and emotionally sober.

As we worked the Steps, our prayer life changed. We prayed for freedom from lust. "At the very beginning, all I could do when the compulsion struck was cry out, 'I'm powerless, please help me'" (*SA* 159). We prayed for those we lusted after: "God bless her and give her what she needs" (*SA* 162). We prayed that true power and love would be demonstrated through us. We prayed for others to receive the blessings of a full life. We prayed that our defects be removed so that we could be more useful to others. We prayed in the morning, in the evening, in the car, on the phone, with laughter, with tears, while listening, while speaking, in silence, aloud. While some people recommended that we begin the day with God and others that we end the day with God, we found that the greatest serenity can be found when we spend the day with God. We strove to live our life as a prayer. Gradually, sometimes haltingly, we were surrendering our will. When we reached Step Eleven, we prayed for the knowledge of God's will for us and the power to carry it out.

In meditation—our time of listening—our purpose was to bring ourselves more fully into harmony with our Higher Power's will for us. We found that meditation was not a single discipline, and there are many ways to listen. Most meditative practices seemed to have in common a quieting of the mind and relaxation of the body. Some of us focused on a particular verse, passage, or visual image, or on our breathing; others let the mind wander and watched where it went. We became more aware of our thoughts, feelings, mental distractions, and emotional discomforts and learned to detach from them.

Often, unexpected answers and options came to us. Even if nothing surfaced or if our thoughts continued to race, we knew that time spent with our Higher Power was helping to build our trust. We let go of our concerns about the day with the expectation that during the day, through many different means, we would receive guidance on how to respond to any situation that arose. It was not necessary to become an expert on meditation; it was only necessary that we make a beginning and continue to practice. Meditation promised to open a great vista of spiritual growth and experience in our lives.

We learned that improving our relationship with God, like continuing to take personal inventory, was a necessary part of the daily maintenance of our recovery. We sought to spend time and attention each day cleaning house (Step Ten), trusting God (Step Eleven), and helping others (Step Twelve). *Alcoholics Anonymous* reminds us that our sobriety depends on it: "What we really have is a daily reprieve contingent on the maintenance of our spiritual condition" (85).

> How fortunate we are, then, to be so needy that we have to find what our lust was really looking for—the loving God who is our refuge and our strength.
>
> ...Our wrongs had separated us, not from praying to God (many of us did that ad nauseam), but from *union* with our God (*SA* 136).

Many of us found it helpful to set aside a regular time, or times, each day for prayer and meditation. Gradually, this discipline became more and more meaningful to us. We also used prayer and meditation at times of stress or when we were triggered by lust or strong emotion. When our petitions grew out of a desire for recovery, we could often see that they were answered. When we were open to receiving guidance and doing God's will, we found more emotional balance. We began to feel that we belonged, that we were part of the universe, and that there was beauty and love for us to give and receive.

But what were we to do when tragedy struck? Some of us hoped that staying sober and trying to do God's will would make us immune from the troubles of the world. Unfortunately, they did not. But they enabled us to see even tragedy in a different light, and brought us, eventually, to a new understanding of God's power to bring joy out of sorrow. Many of us have found

> . . . that out of every season of grief or suffering, when the hand of God seemed heavy or even unjust, new lessons for living were learned, new resources of courage were uncovered, and that finally, inescapably, the conviction came that God *does* "move in a mysterious way His wonders to perform" (*12&12* 105).

The list of demands that had been our previous prayer life was being replaced by an attitude of prayerful acceptance. With this new attitude, even the ordinary common events of our day took on new meaning. Our actions began to lose their selfish motivation and gain spiritual significance. As prayer and meditation became more and more a part of our lives, we noticed that we were living from the heart rather than from the head. We genuinely appreciated opportunities to be helpful to others. We found joy in the happiness of others. "We were learning how to give; and the measure we gave was the measure we got back" (*SA* 62).

> Perhaps one of the greatest rewards of meditation and prayer is the sense of *belonging* that comes to us. We no longer live in a completely hostile world. We are no longer lost and frightened and purposeless. The moment we catch even a glimpse of God's will, the moment we begin to see truth, justice, and love as the real and eternal things in life, we are no longer deeply disturbed by all the seeming evidence to the contrary that surrounds us in purely human affairs. We know that God lovingly watches over us. We know that when we turn to Him, all will be well with us, here and hereafter. (*12&12* 105)

## *Members of SA Share*

*1*

My sponsor told me two things about the Eleventh Step. First, he said it's not prayer *or* meditation—it's prayer *and* meditation. Which means I practice both. Second, he explained to me that he couldn't tell me what meditation is, but he could tell me what it's not. Meditation is not about me. It's about getting rid of me in my head, and making some space for God.

I was taught to start slowly. At first, I meditated for no more than one minute each morning. After a while, I increased it to two. Currently I try to meditate for five to ten minutes in the morning.

I began to just sit and try to watch my thoughts go by. As soon as one thought left, another popped in. Gradually, I began to notice a tiny little space in between the thoughts. Just a moment of silence would pass before another thought barged in, and getting those little bits of quiet did wonders for me. Little by little, those moments of silence became longer. I was creating more space in my head for God, and I have learned in my recovery that less of me and more of my Higher Power is a very good thing.

*2*

Early in recovery, in order to stay sober, I began to recite the first three Steps, the Serenity Prayer, and the Third Step Prayer before I got out of bed in the morning. I kept program literature at my bedside and read it each morning.

This simple morning routine had a dramatic effect on my life. Taking time to remember who I was, that I had a Higher Power, and that I was not in charge, changed my attitude toward the people and events of my life. Spending a few minutes to "think about the twenty-four hours ahead" (*AA* 86) reduced my stress and agitation. I began to experience more emotional balance, better sleep, and smoother relationships.

I consciously began to remind myself during the day that I was a sexaholic and I was powerless over lust. When disturbed I would repeat the Serenity Prayer and close with "Thy will be done." Sometimes I would recite Step Eleven, asking for knowledge of

God's will for me and the power to carry it out.

I did this all for my own survival. Though I didn't realize it at the time, I had made a simple beginning on Step Eleven. Later, when working this Step, I expanded my morning routine to include more reading and prayer and a more structured meditation practice. As my relationship with my Higher Power continues to grow, my other relationships improve along with it.

*3*

For a while before recovery, with self-centered motives, I compulsively practiced various forms of meditation. Each time, when my problems failed to go away, I stopped the practice, thinking it was just another failed technique.

When in sobriety I came to Step Eleven, I began to see that the problem was not the technique—it was that I was bent on doing my will, which is always a recipe for disaster. Instead, I began to pray for God's will for me and the power to carry it out.

I began to have a new experience. I began to have intuitive feelings about what to do in difficult situations. I began to see how I could be part of the solution in everyday matters, often by staying out of them and letting them work themselves out. I began to see that a heart-to-heart talk with my spouse or my child could be a form of meditation. My personality began to soften. Once again, I found God doing for me what I could not do for myself (*AA* 84).

*4*

I was newly sober, on the road, and triggered by lust. I made some phone calls, connected with my sponsor, and the craving passed.

Today, my spiritual toolbox is with me every day wherever I go. I could not be sober without spending time with my Higher Power in the morning. My few minutes of prayer have grown to a thirty-minute time of meditation, spiritual reading, and prayer. I call at least two people from the program every day to maintain serenity. I know that the longer I am in recovery and the more open I am to the wisdom of the fellowship and my sponsor, the more tools I will add to my toolbox. I am so grateful for these! My sobriety—and therefore my life—depend on them.

*5*

My relationship with God was colored by my religious experience growing up. I didn't speak King James English, and it never occurred to me that God might be bilingual. I didn't think prayer would work for me because it seemed too formal.

My sponsor suggested that I begin to talk with God the way I talked with him. He gave me permission to swear, tell jokes, laugh, and cry with God. I was a little tentative with this new idea at first, but it began to grow on me. Before long God and I were buddies. Over time I have grown to be able to have regular prayer time and to sit quietly in His presence, but we still know how to have fun together too.

*6*

Praying for my own selfish desires before recovery brought me no serenity, but instead reinforced my self-pity and self-centered fear. The time I spend praying for the welfare of others has a very different effect on me.

In SA, I have been taught to pray for others: those I lusted after, those I resented, and those I wanted to help. While I am sure God does not need my direction in order to care for others, I find that *I benefit from directing my good will toward them*. Praying for others replaces my self-pity and self-centered fear with loving-kindness.

*7*

When I came to Step Eleven, I balked. With family, work, and a full life, I did not see how I could find time for regular prayer and meditation. I called my sponsor, ready to quit the program. She suggested that I go back to Step Ten to find what was keeping me from moving forward.

I found that I had some rigid ideas about how to work Step Eleven, and I was afraid that I would not be able to do it *right*. I thought I had to do certain morning and evening routines, and I was afraid I would not be able to perform as I *should*. I was afraid of commitment to that discipline. Just as I was afraid of intimacy in all my relationships, I was afraid of intimacy with my Higher Power. Fear and perfectionism—it was time to let go of them.

Asking for God's will for me, I gave myself the freedom to create my own Eleventh Step practice. I discovered that I had to look at *all* of my day as prayer and meditation. I had to regard my entire life as a sacred experience. It was not about getting it right twice a day—*or ever*. For me, it was about approaching life with a different attitude.

I also realized that I had to change my conception of God. When I began to regard Her as a guiding, caring friend and companion, intimacy no longer seemed threatening.

*8*

It is a miracle that I found a God of my understanding, the God who loved me so much that He brought me to this wonderful fellowship of Sexaholics Anonymous. My God is my good friend today. I can talk to Him any time or place. I occasionally lapse back into the belief in a God of retribution who is out to get me. When that happens I ask God to remove that thought from me and I am reminded of how much He loves me. How do I stay sober today? It is simple. I do the same things that worked for me when I first came into the program. I get on my knees each morning and evening to give my Higher Power my day. I pray for His will for me.

## *Step into Action*
### *Recommended Readings*

We suggest that members read and study the following before working the Step:

*Alcoholics Anonymous* (*AA*)
Chapter Six 85–88

*Sexaholics Anonymous* (*SA*)
Step Eleven 135–41

*Twelve Steps and Twelve Traditions* (*12&12*)
Step Eleven 96–105

## *One Method of Working Step Eleven*

Morning routines vary among members, but often include contemplation of at least the first three Steps: we remember that we are sexaholics, we remember that we have a new relationship with a benevolent Higher Power, and we reaffirm our decision to turn our will and lives over to the care of God, as we understand God. We usually include prayers and readings from SA, AA, and other spiritual or religious literature. We take quiet time to contemplate our reading, to consider our options for the day, and to review our emotional condition and surrender any lust. We may share with those close to us, our sponsor, our spouse (not our lust temptations, of course), or an SA friend. We may include specific meditative or religious practices. We ask God for one more day of sobriety. We ask God to direct our thoughts and actions. We ask for God's guidance and power to handle each situation.

While most of us spend some quiet time each morning and evening, we can also find quiet time during lunch or at any other time of day. We may meditate more than once a day if we are able. We seek to establish a daily discipline. As in other areas of our recovery, we discover that we benefit from having a routine. The positive effects of prayer and meditation, hearing God's will and accepting the power to carry it out, motivate us to do more.

Meditation, like any other skill, requires practice. There are many books on meditation, and many methods to choose from. We may seek suggestions from religious and spiritual teachers, our sponsor, and our fellows in recovery. We may wish to attend classes and retreats to learn about meditation.

We take God with us as we go through our day, often expressing gratitude and noting specific things for which we are thankful. Some of us imagine carrying a direct communication line to God, walking hand-in-hand with our Higher Power, or being in the presence of God. We encounter many opportunities each day to send up a prayer or to take a few moments to quiet down. Our prayers are frequent, and can be as short as "Thanks!" or "Help!" or they can be lengthy conversations as time permits.

We learn to pause during the day, when unsure, and renew our request for knowledge of God's will for us and the power to carry it out. A simple prayer or repetition of a verse can have wonderful effects on our attitude and our ability to deal with the world. Some of us carry program literature or a small card with a prayer or slogan to read in times of distress. We put the Serenity Prayer on our computers as a screen saver or set our watch or cell phone to beep periodically, reminding us to practice the presence of God. We ask for guidance, for our Higher Power's will for us. This is how we align our will with God's. This is "the proper use of the will" (*AA* 85).

Perhaps we are unsure whether we have been guided by our own selfish will. Here we find it useful to follow three simple guidelines. First, we continue to pray for God's guidance and for the open-mindedness and willingness to receive it. Second, we share our ideas and progress with our sponsor, other sober members, trusted friends, or spiritual advisors. Third, we take time to pray before making important decisions. We give up our impulsive demand for immediate action and practice patience.

Later in the day, another period of meditation or prayer can help us relax and let go of tension and adjust our attitude. A good time to do this is at the end of our workday, on our evening commute, or before dinner.

At day's end we take time for a thoughtful review. We thank God for the events and lessons of the day, for our sobriety and other blessings. We ask to be kept safe and free from lust during the night. We ask to be kept sober so that we may continue to be helpful to others.

> In times of great stress, situations may threaten to overwhelm us and God may seem far away. Although it may be a challenge that will cause growth in our recovery, even the simplest prayer can become laborious. The White Book offers a special prayer for such difficult times:
>
> > Thus, every problem, no matter how small or great; every crisis, resentment, pain, illness, stress, conflict, depression—any and all of them, without exception—can be turned into good. Every time we feel overwhelmed, our sponsor can point the

> way out of self-pity, resentment, or fear and onto right thinking, helping us say, *"I thank God for the good and the seemingly bad as necessary for my growth. Thy will, not mine, be done"* (*SA* 74 - 75).

We practice prayer and meditation in order to align our will more closely with God's. As we find the power to carry out God's will, we begin to see more opportunities to be of service. We begin to see how we can carry the message of our recovery. We begin to see how the principles of recovery can apply to other areas of our lives. These new ideas add up to a mounting awareness of God working in our lives: a spiritual awakening. This awakening brings us to Step Twelve.

> The essence of Step Eleven is letting God in through every temptation, emotion, difficulty, success, failure, sadness, and joy. True union with the source of our lives (*SA* 141).

## *Some Questions to Consider*

1. What preconceptions have I had about prayer? About meditation?
2. Am I open to asking my Higher Power to guide me in my practice of Step Eleven? How has my Higher Power guided me? How do I pray and meditate?
3. What, for me, is conscious contact with God?
4. How have I been mistaken about God's will for me in the past? How has my understanding of God's will for me changed as I have worked the Steps?
5. What is the value of following God's will for me?
6. Have I had the experience of accepting the power to carry it out? What can I do to become more open to that experience?
7. How has Step Eleven changed my prayer life?
8. What action am I willing to take to practice prayer and meditation?
9. How can I make a beginning on that today?
10. Is my prayer and meditation practiced throughout the day? How might that happen?

## *Step Twelve*

*Having had a spiritual awakening as the result of these steps, we tried to carry this message to sexaholics and to practice these principles in all our affairs.*

In Step Twelve, the cumulative power of working the Twelve Steps entered into every aspect of our lives. Awakened spiritually, we were moved to share what we had discovered with others. And as we did so we found—with deep wonder and gratitude—what we had been looking for in lust all along.

> We are filled in the giving. . . .
> . . . All along, this is what we had really been looking for, lusting for, sexing for, and taking for. By taking, we had separated ourselves from others, ourselves, and God. By giving, we found true union with others and God, and, lo and behold, love itself. But it slipped in unrecognized through the back door. "Surprised by joy" *SA* 148).

### *A Spiritual Awakening*

When we first read Step Twelve, the idea of a spiritual awakening did not seem all that important. Most of us just wanted some relief from the problem. We were not focused on, and sometimes not even interested in, a spiritual life. But as we began to participate in the Fellowship and to work the Steps, we were unable to explain what was keeping us sexually sober. Most of us had thought we would never be able to surrender our lust. Yet, with time and practice, we found ourselves able to surrender more easily and gracefully. We noticed that other areas of our life seemed to be improving as well. Although we could not explain *how* it worked, as long as it kept working we would continue following instructions. Working the first eleven Steps in order, with the guidance of an SA sponsor, set the stage for a personality change sufficient to overcome sexaholism, that is, a spiritual awakening:

> Spiritual awakening is not mere sobriety, an awakening to knowledge about the Steps, belief in the Steps, or psychological insights into why they work. It is a change of state, an awakening of what was once dead (*SA* 144).

A spiritual awakening amounts to a new state of consciousness and a realization of new power: we find ourselves able to do what was once beyond our strength.

> When a man or a woman has a spiritual awakening, the most important meaning of it is that he has now become able to do, feel, and believe that which he could not do before on his unaided strength and resources alone. He has been granted a gift which amounts to a new state of consciousness and being.... In a very real sense he has been transformed. . . . He finds himself in possession of a degree of honesty, tolerance, unselfishness, peace of mind, and love of which he had thought himself quite incapable. What he has received is a free gift, and yet usually, at least in some small part, he has made himself ready to receive it (*12&12* 106-7).

By the time we arrived at Step Twelve, we had discovered gratitude and serenity. We had a new attitude toward life, seeing it as purposeful and rewarding. We had developed depth of character and faith that supported us through difficult times with unfamiliar serenity. Instead of being slaves to our feelings, we became able to maintain an "emotional sobriety" that we had never known. It was no longer faith in our own strength or abilities that sustained us, but faith in a Power greater than ourselves. It was not faith that our life would be problem free, but rather that we would be given whatever we needed to deal with our problems. We trusted that we would learn what we needed to learn and that ultimately, all would be well. We no longer believed we needed to control the outcome of a situation, but instead found faith that no matter what happened, we would be all right. We placed less importance on trusting the people in our lives and instead learned to trust a benevolent Higher Power that works through people and situations. This faith gave us the courage we needed to face life on life's terms.

### *Carrying the Message*

We awoke to a new awareness: we had a message to carry, and a responsibility to carry it. We had found a solution that required only the working of twelve simple Steps within a Fellowship of sobriety. This solution was freely given to us, and to keep it alive for ourselves, we had to pass it on to others.

We told our stories and shared the SA solution without being invested in the results. We were responsible for carrying the message, not the sexaholic. We remembered that Step 12 states only that we *tried* to carry this message. We were not responsible for whether or not others accepted the message of recovery. Nor were we responsible for another person's ability to get or stay sober. That was between them and their Higher Power.

We accepted that we have a solution. We don't claim that it's for everyone, but for us it works. Nonetheless, in spite of the questions, struggles, and confusion that we have gone through, we find that sexual sobriety is truly the key to a happy and joyous freedom we could otherwise never know. SA is not for everyone who needs it; SA is for those who want it. Nor do we claim that sobriety alone will lead to a lasting and joyous recovery (*SA* 2).

We who had spent our lives in hiding now opened ourselves to fellowship. As others had done for us, we reached out to newcomers with a message of hope. We participated in SA meetings, where we shared the solution with others. We volunteered for service positions in our group. We sponsored others. We served at local, regional, and international levels. We took SA into prisons and treatment centers. We wrote for SA publications and corresponded with loners and imprisoned members. We helped organize regional and international conferences. As we participated in service work and learned to cooperate with other sexaholics, we experienced a new joy and spiritual growth. We found great satisfaction in giving without expecting anything in return. And we found our solution at last in being useful to God and others.

*In All Our Affairs*

The Steps had changed our lives by making recovery from lust possible. We grew in recovery by applying the principles embodied in the Steps to other areas of our lives. We surrendered strained relations with our spouse, children, boss, or co-workers to God. We took personal inventories, surrendered our shortcomings, and made amends, first with regard to lust and eventually in every area of our lives.

Practicing the principles, we found ourselves less likely to be concerned with the faults of others. Instead, we kept the focus on our own shortcomings and admitted our own wrongs. In so doing, our behavior and our attitudes changed. Inside and outside of SA, we found the freedom to accept others as they were. As we practiced accepting ourselves and others, we wasted less energy obsessing about how things ought to be.

We also began to apply the principle of service to other areas of our lives. We looked for opportunities to share our time, patience, understanding, and compassion, and to serve others at work, at home, and elsewhere. We who had been driven by selfishness and self-seeking, were learning the simple joys of service.

The Steps had taught us to relate responsibly with others and showed us that service was the path to serenity and true happiness. We now saw that we could actually help to make the world a better place. As instruments of peace, harmony, and goodwill, we gave back out of the abundance we had received. We tried to carry the message of SA recovery to other sexaholics. We reached out to others and practiced the principles of the program in our relations with the wider world. The Twelfth Step became a plan for living the rest of our lives.

> We began practicing a positive sobriety, taking the actions of love to improve our relations with others. We were learning how to give; and the

> measure we gave was the measure we got back. We were finding what none of the substitutes had ever supplied. We were making the real Connection. We were home (*SA* 62).

> *The only thing I can bear witness to is the truth of my own experience. Because that's what I want to hear from others. I want to see and feel the real truth about someone's inner life and behavior that I can identify with.*
> *. . . Coming to see and acknowledge the truth about myself is what got me through the door into this new way of life. It's the truth about myself—the imperfect truth—that attracts others; not all the preaching in the world (SA* 144*).*

## *Members of SA Share*

### *1*

I got involved in service work for an entirely selfish reason—my sponsor told me that service would strengthen my recovery. So I volunteered to take over a service position from my sponsor—leading newcomer orientation meetings. I also attended intergroup meetings and volunteered to take the minutes and hold service positions. I began to sponsor others—helping them work the Steps, listening to their struggles and victories, and sharing my own. From time to time they have called me on my character defects, and I have made amends to them. I have tried to share my life with them.

As it turned out, my sponsor was right: getting involved in service greatly increased my willingness to practice the Steps, and made my life and attitudes less burdensome to me. I got a tremendous amount of help and motivation by making myself as accountable to those I sponsored as they were to me. Service has taken me out of myself and my problems. It has put me in contact with members from other parts of the U.S. and other countries. I have benefited by corresponding with people in recovery in places such as Russia, Singapore, Australia, China, and Ireland.

Step Twelve has been a great gift to the quality of my life and my recovery. Without the SA program, I would never have been able to receive or even want that gift.

*2*

My home group meeting is the highlight of my week. Home group members arrive twenty minutes early to set up chairs and tables and greet all who attend. We take great care to ensure that the meeting reflects the solution. After the meeting we usually have coffee and brownies, and hang around talking to newcomers.

We've worked hard over the years to make the meeting a place where sobriety can happen, so that the meeting itself becomes a vehicle for Twelfth Step work. For three weeks every summer, we read *Practical Guidelines for Group Recovery* to gauge how healthy our group is; it's our way of doing a group inventory. Last time we read it, one long-term member commented, "It feels really good to say that this group does everything that's recommended in that pamphlet."

While I sponsor people and share on the phone between meetings, I believe my most effective Twelfth Step work is done right at the home group. Whether I'm doing my service job, sharing my experience in the meeting, or talking to a suffering member afterwards, it's a chance to spread the message of SA and give back a little of what I've been given.

*3*

My sponsor told me I had two choices: I could either carry the message or I could set it down. I had come a long way up from my bottom, and I knew that dropping this life-saving message was not an option for me.

So, I would start to be active in service after my life stabilized, and I had everything together. But it turned out that I had it backwards. It was as I followed my sponsor's example and began to serve that I felt better and my life improved.

*4*

A friend in my church group introduced me to the man who became my first sponsor. We communicated with the help of a computer because he did not know sign language at all. Even with his help, it took eight months for me to get to attend the SA meeting because I needed a sign language interpreter to participate in the meeting. At first the group was worried about hiring interpreters, who were not members, to come to a closed meeting. Once they understood the code of ethics among certified interpreters, which emphasizes confidentiality, they were willing to give it a try.

In the meeting, I immediately felt I was home. I was grateful that there was a holy place for me to be with other sexaholics and share experience, strength, and hope. I carried the message to some other people in the deaf community, and now we are three. Other members have remarked that they are glad to have deaf members among them because our stories help them to stay sober. My shame and guilt eventually turned to humility and serenity.

What has been working for me is to go to meetings, share my story, see my sponsor regularly, pray and meditate, serve as a coffee maker and librarian, sponsor a deaf man, attend other interpreted Twelve Step meetings, and chair a marathon meeting. The tools I have learned in SA have helped me to enjoy being a deacon in my church, a college professor, and an actor. Most importantly, the tools have helped me enjoy being myself.

I want to reach out to SA members across the nation and around the world, especially to other deaf SA members. I pray that someday I will have access to SA meetings in other towns or at regional conferences and international conventions.

Today I feel calm, delighted, and hopeful. I know that I do not have to run away or find instant sexual gratification. My Higher Power is with me and so is my SA Fellowship.

*5*

I began to participate in taking meetings to a long-term drug and alcohol treatment center. Few of the clients had ever considered or even heard of sexaholism. As we told our stories, I watched understanding dawn in their eyes. Several of them began to identify with us: "Oh no, that's me too!" Some shared that their inability to stay clean and sober from drugs and alcohol was due to their lusting. Although some were discouraged at the prospect of having to consider yet another addiction, they began to have hope. They could see our recovery and our freedom and began to believe that they could have that too. I have not forgotten the warmth of that experience of sharing hope where there was none. That is both the fuel and the fruit of my recovery.

*6*

My recovery did not feel complete. One day, a plea went out of my heart to God, saying, "There must be some useful purpose, some other work you want me to do besides supporting my immediate family." Minutes later I got a telephone call from an SA member asking if I would be interested in doing prison service work. I couldn't believe it, yet it was clearly the next right thing. I felt like it was what God wanted me to do.

I have since become involved in writing and sending out literature to inmates, sponsoring inmates, sponsoring an SA group in prison, and encouraging other members who want to do similar service work. I am thankful to be part of lifesaving and life-changing work. It's a gift to feel useful.

*7*

One year, no one from my group was willing to serve as our intergroup representative. I am so grateful that I took it on. For two years I participated in the regional assembly, took the minutes, and even brought a motion from my intergroup. I was almost ready to rotate off when the Delegate stepped down. Again, no one else was willing to serve and I was elected as an Assembly Delegate representing my region.

It was a thrill for me to take a place at the table of the General Delegate Assembly (GDA). There was plenty of work to do. Currently, I serve on two Trustee committees and participate in teleconferences one or two days per month.

I had already studied the Steps and Traditions, but as a Delegate, I learned about the Twelve Concepts for World Service. I learned that, in the inverted pyramid of service, the ultimate authority resides in the groups (Concept One), but that that authority is "delegated" to trusted servants (Concept Two). As a Delegate, I served as part of the "active voice and the effective conscience" of the fellowship. I also learned that I was endowed with the "Right of Decision" (Concept Three), which means I had to vote my conscience. So while I considered the wishes of my region, and listened carefully to the opinions of my colleagues in the GDA, no one dictated my vote. I must stay sober and spiritually fit, so that I can leave the channel open for guidance from my Higher Power.

Much of my work was done in my own region. I traveled to regional gatherings when I could, and stayed in touch with the Intergroup Representatives (IGR) by phone. We began to develop a network of Group Service Representatives (GSR) so that all groups will be represented and unified in our service structure. It is my hope that if I do my part, someday our region will be like a well-tuned instrument, where every chord vibrates in harmonious unity.

*8*

I know today that I am blessed to be in prison and alive. If I hadn't been sent here I would probably be dead because this is where I found SA. So I thank my Higher Power for locking me up. God took me, an otherwise useless old thing, and gave me a purpose for being alive. I could feel sorry for myself, but when I try to carry the message of sobriety and see people get into the program and stay sober, I feel good about myself.

Most of the men in my group are serving long term sentences, and we are interested in learning how other members recover. We have been fortunate to have contact with SA members from the outside. Over the years several members of the SA Correctional Facilities Committee have visited me and showed me how to stay sober and work the Steps.

I am not a well-educated person, but I believe that I can give moral support to people who want to stop lusting and live productive, happy lives. I carry the message as much as I can by mail to help me stay sober. I correspond with other SA members in prison and on the outside, and I tell them I would be glad to walk the path of recovery with them. I find that the more I give the program away to others, the stronger I become in my own recovery.

My Higher Power has given me a very peaceful way to live in a place where very few people can find serenity. As I serve out my life sentence, carrying the SA message gives purpose to my everyday life. I have come to believe that is why my Higher Power has shown me how to enjoy a sober and stable life.

*9*

Practicing these principles in all my affairs is proving to be a wonderful way to live. One of the first ways I did this was to apply the Twelve Traditions to my workplace and my relationships there. What a concept! Then I noticed that my eating behaviors were compulsive at times, and I had to ask myself why I eat what I ate, and if the portions were appropriate. For me, this did not require working all Twelve Steps on food, but for many others I know it has. Currently, I am unofficially working the Steps on my codependence. By unofficially, I mean that I have not joined another fellowship nor found a sponsor in that fellowship, but I discuss my codependent behaviors with my SA sponsor (who has worked a co-dependent's program). I realize I am powerless over what other people think of me. It is none of my business what other people think of me. What other people think of me should not be a factor in my life decisions. I have to seek the will of my Higher Power, and make decisions to align my behavior with God's will. Other people's opinions are just that—opinions, and none of my business.

*10*

In my fifth year of sobriety I received the gift of an exciting career change with challenging leadership responsibilities. Brought in to my organization as an agent of change, I have to work with many colleagues who are very happy with the status quo. What a surprise to learn that their resistance to my "great ideas" would touch my character defects—like feeling less than. I am so grateful that when I find that I am less than kind, over-passionate, over-powering, or just less effective than I would like to be, I can make an immediate public amends (Step 10) and refocus the meeting. I am also learning that surrendering my character defects prior to the meeting (Seventh Step Prayer) and recommitting to my Higher Power (Third Step Prayer) prior to a difficult meeting greatly increases the probability of a successful meeting. Afterwards I give gratitude for having been useful to others (Step 12). I would never have stepped up to this position without this Program and the Steps.

### *11*

One of the first three things my sponsor told me to do is read the AA *Big Book*—two to four pages a day, and when I'm done, start over. I get through the basic text three or four times each year, and I often marvel at how some words I read before have new meaning to me the next time through.

The most profound re-read was after I had made most of my amends and was sponsoring fellow sexaholics. It occurred to me that every description of what the people who wrote the Big Book said of their experience as the result of working the Twelve Steps matched my experience exactly! I did what they said they did, and I got what they said they got. Now, when I read "we" in the Big Book, I include myself in unity with the first hundred.

I tell my sponsees not to want what I have, but what the first hundred told us they got. And if the sponsees decide they want the results described in the Big Book, I can guarantee they will have it by doing what the authors did.

### *12*

It was not difficult for me to see how the wisdom of the program principle, "surrender to God what I cannot fight with my own power, and let His power fight my temptations" could be applied in all areas of my life. But it was not so easy to practice this principle in all the areas of my life.

Lust, acting-out, and addiction had brought me to my knees in the First Step. It took time for me to realize that only that First Step experience could give me the willingness to surrender the constant resentments that always led to fights with my wife.

Practicing this principle of surrender was the only hope to heal our marriage and bring back the kind of relationship we had hoped for in the beginning.

I also had to apply Program principles in my professional life. It took me time to realize that I was powerless over the many problems of my clients. I started praying for these clients and their problems, and I surrendered them to God. This brought astounding results in many cases, and it saved my serenity and nerves more than I can say.

*13*

I may not be the best person to judge whether I've had a spiritual awakening or not, since I believed I was spiritually fit in my pre-SA life. I take it as a good sign, though, that people tell me they're happy when I'm around. People didn't often say that before.

I know I'm no longer "spiritually asleep" to the fact that my acting out is destructive. As a fellow SA joked, "The program hasn't cured me, but it's ruined acting out for me forever."

I've been sober for almost two years now, and even—God forbid—if I were to slip, I'm no longer asleep to the fact that there is a solution and that it can work for me.

*14*

I'm starting to see how I can practice the principles of the Steps in daily living.

As a principle of Step Two, I believe a power greater than me restores me to sanity through friends and advisors in and outside of SA. In consideration of the Fifth Step, I share about my defects in discussions with family and friends. Many have shared that this honesty has helped them with problems in their own lives.

As a principle of Step Ten, I try to go through the day open to the possibility that my ideas might be wrong or incomplete and that I require the perspective of others. Step Eleven comes to mind when I try to be a channel of peace to others.

*15*

Coming out of the SA International Convention in Detroit, I

felt the need to connect daily in an intentional way with those I sponsor and others who I work with regularly in their recovery. I enjoy writing and, although I often procrastinate, have benefitted greatly by writing my inventories. In mid-July I began sending a daily group text message to seven people with whom I either have a sponsorship or accountability relationship. As I daily shared my experience, strength and hope some amazing things started to happen! First, my own recovery and connection with God started to take off as I wrote about my continued struggles with resentment and fear and the victory I was gaining as I surrendered to God through the application of the Twelve Steps. I also started receiving positive feedback from those who were receiving the texts. Some individuals asked if they could forward the messages to others. My sponsor encouraged me to begin submitting these messages for possible inclusion in the SA Meditations book and *Essay*. In the past month and a half my personal group text list has grown to 18 people with many of these people forwarding these messages to others. The circle keeps growing! I have no idea how many people are reading these messages, but I know that others are being helped and growing in their recovery because I have humbled myself and become willing to share my experience, strength, and hope from the vantage point of my weaknesses and, by the grace of God, victories.

In addition, I am experiencing personal growth as a result. I am growing in joy, peace, and hope. My fears are being confronted on a regular basis and are being consistently overcome! I am making amends that I never thought I could. My relationship and level of intimacy with my wife and family is stronger than ever. My connection with God is genuine and intimate as I am learning to trust Him like I never have before. I have always believed in the importance of 12th Step work to individual and group recovery, but as I have stepped out in faith and gone against my fears God is doing in and through me more than I could have ever dreamed! All things are possible as we trust in God and become willing to give it all away!

## *Step into Action*

### *Recommended Readings*

We suggest that members read and study the following before working the Step:

*Alcoholics Anonymous* (*AA*)
"Working with Others" 89-103
Appendix II 567-68

*Sexaholics Anonymous* (*SA*)
"Step Twelve" 143-55
"Starting a New SA Group" 173-84
"Meetings—How They Work" 185-9

*Twelve Steps and Twelve Traditions* (*12&12*)
"Step Twelve" 106-125

## *One Method of Working Step Twelve*

> ...The joy of living is the theme of A.A.'s [SA's]* Twelfth Step, and action is the key word. Here we begin to practice all Twelve Steps of the program in our daily lives so that we and those about us may find emotional sobriety (*12 x 12* 106).

We took action. We worked the Steps. We stayed sexually sober. We confronted our fears, shared our secrets, and made amends. We had been incapable of this before recovery. Not only have we been freed from the obsession with lust and the compulsion to act out sexually, we have also begun to view life in a new way.

The change in our lives has been dramatic. As the result of working Steps One through Eleven, we have had a spiritual awakening, a "personality change sufficient to bring about recovery" (*AA* 567). Step 12 states that this spiritual awakening is "the" result of working the Steps—not just "a" result. This new relationship with a Higher Power, this "faith that works" (as Bill W. of AA called it), is what guides and directs our thinking and behavior and empowers us to live free of the tyranny of lust.

Our spiritual awakening propels us to carry the message to the sexaholic who still suffers. This gift of sobriety and recovery was freely given to us, and it is our responsibility to pass it on to those who need it. Indeed, we discover that in order to keep it we must give it away. This is the essence of carrying the message: one sexaholic to another, we continue to share our spiritual awakening.

We cannot give away what we do not have so we must continue to live according to the principles of our newfound life, and we continue to work the Steps with a sponsor. After working Step Twelve, some members return to Step One and repeat the process, while others focus on Steps Ten, Eleven, and Twelve. The important thing is to continue—for ourselves and for those around us.

Even before we reach Step Twelve, we are already carrying the message in many ways. We attend meetings. We share our stories. We listen to others. We make and receive phone calls on a daily basis. We give others rides to meetings. We make coffee, set up chairs, and clean up after gatherings. We participate in fellowship outside of meetings. We work the Steps and share the solution.

When we meet newcomers, we take time to welcome them into the Fellowship. We listen to their stories and tell them ours. We answer questions about SA as best we can. We give them a phone list and introduce them to other members. Often we take their phone number and call them in the days following their first meeting just to keep in touch.

One of the most important ways that we work Step Twelve is to make ourselves available to sponsor other members. This sacred relationship between sponsor and sponsee provides a vehicle for us to pass along the wisdom we received from the Fellowship and the recovery we received from our Higher Power. We simply share our experiences in working the Steps—what worked for us and what *didn't* work for us. Using resources like this book, we work through the Steps again, alongside of our sponsee–guiding, encouraging, suggesting, discussing, exhorting, and loving them as led by God.

In addition to working with newcomers and sponsees, we continue to share our experience, strength, and hope with accountability partners, recovery friends, sponsor, and other members of Sexaholics Anonymous. We respond to phone calls and meet with members to provide assistance whenever we are able, knowing that we benefit as well. We share honestly what has worked for us. When appropriate, we encourage others to seek opportunities for service. We stress that action is the key to joyous recovery.

We have learned that self-centeredness has been a primary cause of our problems, and that helping others brings us not only recovery but also real joy. When we share the SA program of recovery with others, we are reminded of the solution. As we practice this "design for living" (*AA* 15), we are able to be of real usefulness in the world and to give back some of what we have received. Performing service to the Fellowship offers rewards beyond our imagination.

Through our Step work, our participation in the Fellowship, and our service, we learn new behavior and begin to have healthy relationships. Step Twelve suggests that we practice these new skills and principles in all areas of our lives. At home and at work, we recognize what we are powerless over and turn it over to God; we inventory ourselves when we feel any loss of serenity; we tell on ourselves to sponsors and recovery partners, revealing our feelings and temptations; we surrender character defects that we see manifesting; we make amends as soon as we realize we have wronged someone; and we model recovery principles to those around us. As a beloved SA pioneer used to say, "Our lives are the only White Book most people will ever read."

We begin to look at all of our interactions with other people as part of our recovery. Rather than resenting or fearing the people we interact with and losing our serenity, we learn to work the program and take the actions of love in all situations. The alternative to seeking serenity in all of our affairs is chaos in our lives, and this can lead us back to active sexaholism. Thus, we learn to practice these principles in all our affairs.

As part of practicing the principles, we begin to study and practice the Twelve Traditions. The Traditions arise from the experience of AA and serve as useful guidelines to ensure the healthy functioning and growth of SA. We find that the principles inherent in the Traditions teach us to promote unity and are applicable to all of our relationships, both inside and outside the Fellowship.

## *Some Questions to Consider*

1. What does "Having a Spiritual Awakening as a result of these steps" mean to me? In what ways have I had a Spiritual Awakening?
2. What can I do to continue my work on the Twelve Steps? What does my sponsor recommend?
3. What does "tried to carry this message to Sexaholics" mean to me?
4. What am I doing to carry the message to the sexaholic who still suffers? What more am I willing to do?
5. What does "practice these principles in all our affairs" mean to me?
6. Is serving others a priority for me? What can I do to keep the focus on my own recovery while performing service? Do I do too much? Too little?
7. Am I willing to sponsor other members? How have I benefited from carrying the message?
8. What principles does this Step refer to? Which of "these principles" have I begun to practice in other areas of my life? What more can I do?
9. How am I a good example to others in the program? In my family? At work?
10. Which service opportunities are available in my area? Which ones does my sponsor recommend for me? (See the Service list in Appendix B.)
11. What has service work taught me about the Twelve Traditions? How can I apply them to my life?

SA's Twelve Steps are a group of principles, spiritual in their nature, which, if practiced as a way of life, can expel the obsession to drink and enable the sufferer to become happily and usefully whole (*12 x 12* 15).

# *Appendix A*

## *Basic Recovery Tools*

As we read recovery literature and work the Steps with our sponsors, we will be introduced to many new terms and concepts. Sponsors will teach the "language of recovery" as well as the tools many of us use to navigate this "Road of Happy Destiny." Some of our Basic Recovery Tools are described below.

### *Meetings and Fellowship*

We often feel very unsure or shy at our first meetings, in addition to being angry that we need to be there. Yet, each time we attend a meeting we hear something that helps us, or we get an opportunity to share that unburdens us. For these reasons it is good to attend meetings daily if possible. Many SA members have a personal rule that if they don't want to go to a meeting, that's exactly the time they most need to go to a meeting. The desire to skip a meeting is usually our addiction at work.

It is suggested that newcomers and those struggling to remain sober attend ninety meetings in ninety days. This is a powerful tool to develop and maintain a focus on sobriety and working the Steps. If there aren't any SA meetings in your area, there will certainly be other open 12 Step recovery meetings to attend. We don't have to identify as anything other than an addict when attending other fellowships. If we are uncomfortable with that, we don't have to identify at all. We can just sit and listen.

We attend SA meetings to share our personal experience, strength, and hope. We share how the Steps and Traditions help our acceptance of life's difficulties. Meetings are not a dumping ground for our problems. They are not a substitute for working the Steps with our sponsor. In meetings we limit our sharing to allow time for everyone to share. We stick to the topic and share only once until everyone has had a chance to share. We are mindful of the fact that we are not really as important to others as we would like to think we are.

As one SA member wrote, attending meetings:

1. Gets us out of our isolation and our heads,
2. Educates us in the principles of the SA Program,
3. Puts us in touch with more experienced members and exposes us to new ideas so that we can begin to change our thinking and behavior,
4. Puts us in touch with newcomers so that we can keep fresh the memory of what our lives were like before sobriety,
5. Allows us to pass on to others what we have been given—the primary purpose of the SA Program and a key to a happy and peaceful sobriety,
6. Relieves the inner pressure of our character defects through the subtle atmosphere of recovery and a Higher Power present at meetings,
7. Gives a message to ourselves that we are choosing recovery,
8. Allows us to participate in the fellowship of the SA Program,
9. Permits sharing and listening to help us learn to relate to others and to understand there are other viewpoints and perspectives beyond our own.

Tradition Twelve guides our behavior within the Fellowship. We put our spiritual principle of anonymity ahead of any personal desires to talk about SA meetings or conversations. We respect each other's anonymity at meetings by not repeating outside the meeting whom we saw or what a particular person said at the meeting. Practicing anonymity in this way benefits us as individuals and as a group by allowing each member to share freely what is really going on and by protecting the group from gossip, cliques, divisiveness, hero-worship, and other negative behaviors. Through this principle we keep the focus on ourselves, speaking only about the ideas of the SA Program as they apply to us in our own lives.

We focus on the message, not the messenger. We place "principles before personalities."

We also practice anonymity in meetings by not inappropriately discussing our occupations, religious leanings, social groups, incomes, membership in other Twelve Step programs, or other outside affiliations. Likewise, if we see someone in a meeting whom we know in another context, we respect their anonymity by not talking about non-Program matters with them at the meeting. When we focus on our similarities, instead of our differences, we share what is in our hearts, unhampered by the ordinary labels, expectations, and roles that identify us in our "outside" lives. We sit in a meeting as equals, having a common sexaholic problem, rather than as persons divided by social rank or skill.

We practice anonymity outside a meeting when we see an SA program friend in a public place. We refrain from saying hello if the situation would require explaining to a third person how we know each other. This is what protecting anonymity means. In a situation where anonymity should be maintained but is not, we call that "breaking anonymity."

We try to practice anonymity in one-on-one conversations with our sponsor or other trusted friend in the SA Program if we need to discuss an issue that involves a third person. By not saying whom we are talking about we keep the focus on ourselves. After all, we are the one having the issue. We offer spiritual protection for the person we're upset with and avoid gossip and criticism. Our discussion can then focus on what we can change—our own attitudes. We are determined to live in the solution, not the problem.

### *Sponsorship*

Getting a sponsor is humbling. Trusting the experience and insights of another sexaholic as we attend SA meetings and go through the Steps can require a big change in our "I can do it myself" attitude. After all, the way we were living our lives and what we thought we knew about recovery is how we got to SA in the first place. Doing without a sponsor is like piloting a ship without a rudder. The sailor is at the mercy of whatever current comes along. We will need more help. Even those with recovery or a sponsor in another Twelve Step program will benefit by getting an SA sponsor. (Indeed, as we cautioned before, an SA sponsor is required to effectively work through this book. For more on this, read Step Two in the White Book)

When choosing a sponsor, the basic rule is we ask someone who is ahead of us in working the Steps, has successful, continuous sobriety, and seems to have recovery that we would like to have for ourselves. Sponsors should have sponsors themselves and attend meetings regularly. Sponsors can guide us to work the Twelve Steps and show us a way of life through example and by taking time to listen and respond.

It is highly recommended that sponsors in SA be of the same gender as those they sponsor. It is good for the sponsee to ask for help, which demonstrates the sponsee's willingness to work the SA Program. We are in touch with our sponsors, seeing them at meetings and calling them regularly, even daily, especially at the beginning. Some of us have successfully worked the Steps with a sponsor who lives in a distant community. We communicate by phone, internet or mail even if we rarely, or never, sit face to face. Members in prison have recovered in this way. Geographic distance doesn't have to be a barrier in spiritual matters if we have willingness.

A sponsor doesn't do the work of our recovery for us and doesn't provide magic answers to our problems. He or she is not our parent, therapist, or religious advisor. Rather, a sponsor shares his or her experience, strength, and hope and points toward the simple kit of spiritual tools the SA Program offers.

In keeping with Tradition Five, working as a sponsor allows us to carry the message and is a special experience not to be missed. Members become sponsors because this helps us stay sober. We have the opportunity to keep the message alive for ourselves. Having a sponsee allows a sponsor to give service and practice detachment. Being a sponsor allows a member to grow through humility, love, and service. When we sponsor others, we practice the Twelfth Step principle that we must give away that which we have been given.

### *Phone Calls to Share with Others*

When we come to SA we will usually hear someone say, "You never have to be alone again." With the secrets and isolation that characterize this addiction, this is quite a promise. One important way to break out of isolation is to use the phone. Initially, we call our sponsors and other sexaholics whenever we are struggling or obsessing about a sobriety matter. Instead of trying to handle anger, stress, lust triggers, or one of the other daily sexaholic challenges by ourselves, we call another sexaholic. We call others to be reminded of the tools of sobriety and recovery. We call because this helps keep the feeling alive that we belong to a community with a common problem and a solution that works. We call whether we "need" to or not, to create a healthy habit, and to keep this communication channel open. When our sobriety is threatened, we pick up the phone and call.

We are discreet when leaving voice messages for other members. It is possible to inadvertently compromise another member's anonymity by leaving a message that someone else may hear. Unless we have permission, we do not mention the name of the program or other information that might lead to awkward questions or curiosity from family members or coworkers. Leaving a first name only and a phone number is a common practice.

### *Using Fellowship Literature*

We practice our recovery on a daily basis. Last week's recovery, we find, is about as useful in keeping us sober in today's moments of temptation as last week's shower keeps us clean today! We learn to practice an attitude of surrender. Part of our daily recovery practice is reading SA literature. We are able to benefit from others' experience and hear the collective wisdom gained by those walking the road of recovery. As we read of others' struggles, successes, and insights, we find encouragement and inspiration. It is useful to set a regular time for daily reading. Reading each morning gives us a new outlook on the day and healthy new ideas to carry with us. Reading before retiring helps us rest more peacefully. During the day it is useful to have some of this literature available to remind us of the principles of sobriety and recovery at times of stress. Fellowship literature can be like meetings or phone calls with a cover. Throughout this book we make recommendations of material to be read while working the Steps.

An SA group's Literature Chairman will have information about books and pamphlets that may help one to advance in sobriety and recovery. Because the SA program is based on the principles of the AA Twelve Step program, all A.A. General Service Conference-approved literature is approved for SA meetings. The texts listed below deserve additional mention here because they form the foundation of the SA program.

### *Sexaholics Anonymous*

*Sexaholics Anonymous* is also called the SA Manual or "The White Book" (because it is usually bound in a plain white cover for anonymity). Based on the principles discovered by recovering alcoholics and first published in the AA *Big Book*, the White Book evolved in the 1980s as a collection of essays and other pieces defining our Fellowship's unique stand on the spiritual nature of lust addiction and recovery through the Twelve Steps. Written by Roy K., the White Book has been affirmed as the first voice of SA recovery by Sexaholics suffering from all forms of sex and lust addiction, from many different backgrounds, cultures, as well as religious and spiritual traditions, and from all around the world. As we say in SA, a meeting based on readings from the White Book has at least one sober voice present!

### *Alcoholics Anonymous*

First published in 1939, *Alcoholics Anonymous* (*AA*) is familiarly and affectionately called "The *Big Book*" because the first edition, printed on cheap (and therefore, thick) paper to save money, was a large tome indeed. This, the basic text of *Alcoholics Anonymous*, provides insight into the disease of alcoholism and introduces and explains the Twelve Steps as a path of recovery. This information is presented in the first 164 pages. The last part presents a number of stories of alcoholics who found sobriety and a way of life in AA.

We sexaholics use the *AA* text extensively in meetings and in working the SA program. The attributes and attitudes associated with alcoholism speak to us tellingly, and we usually identify with the stories. In the Big Book's explanation of the Twelve Steps is the framework for our program and the solution to our problem.

### *Essay*

*Essay* is the Fellowship's newsletter, appropriately referred to as "our meeting in print." Begun in 1981 as a letter from the SA Central Office to a fledgling membership in widely separated locations at that time, it became a quarterly publication in booklet form in the mid-eighties. In its pages, Fellowship business, a calendar of events, drafts of proposed SA literature, news of SA groups from around the world, member stories, and articles of general interest about recovery written by members can be found. Publications such as *Essay* or *AA Grapevine*, can be carried in a purse, pocket, or briefcase to be read at any convenient time.

In 2004, a decade of articles from *Essay* was collected in book form as *Practical Recovery Tools, 1994-2003*. It is often called "The Yellow Book" for the color of its cover. Written by members for the Fellowship, it offers our collective experience on topics of vital interest.

### *Twelve Steps and Twelve Traditions*

*Twelve Steps and Twelve Traditions*, also called "The *12 & 12*," was written by AA co-founder Bill W. and first published in 1952. These inspiring essays on the Twelve Steps have been put into practice successfully by generations of recovering alcoholics as well as by recovering addicts of various persuasions and fellowships, also with proven success. These essays also serve as the foundational documents for SA's Steps. The 12 & 12's descriptions of the Twelve Steps are longer and more detailed than those in the Big Book. Its essays of the Traditions are rich with examples from the experience of those who got sober early in AA history, as they implemented the principles that would help the fellowship to survive and grow.

### *Prayer*

Prayer is an essential part of our daily routine and sobriety maintenance. There are many ways and reasons to pray. Morning and evening prayer routines help us stay sober daily. We pray for help in becoming the people we believe God wants us to be, following the principles of selflessness outlined in the Third Step Prayer. Many of us pray for our families, friends, and other recovering individuals. We pray when we are triggered by lust or difficult emotions. We use written, memorized, and spontaneous prayers. Prayers may be a sigh, one word, or lengthy ruminations. Prayer draws our attention to the God of our understanding. It is useful to ask God to be with us. Our prayers may look like meditation, dedication, or a walk in the woods. Prayers of gratitude keep us from self-pity or resentment. When we pray, we access the infinite, a benign Power far greater than ourselves, who is ready to help us.

Throughout the SA program we find prayers. While only Step Eleven refers to prayer directly, there are commonly used prayers associated with Steps Three, Four, Seven, and Eleven. In SA we also often use the Serenity Prayer. The text of *Alcoholics Anonymous* includes several formal prayers and numerous instructions to "Ask God" in various situations. In a global Fellowship like SA, prayers come from many cultures, languages, and faith practices.

Sexaholics frequently find memorizing prayers is helpful. When we know a prayer well we can replace lust images and the usual negative or obsessive thoughts with a positive spiritual message. *Twelve Steps and Twelve Traditions* suggests that the only persons who doubt the power of prayer are those who do not do enough of it. That is our experience, too.

### *Working the Steps*

This brings us to the point of this book. The key to the happy, joyous, and free way of life that the SA Program promises is working the Steps. Working the Steps refers to following the guidelines for recovery set out in the Twelve Steps of SA. Step work requires spending time and effort on each of these twelve stages of our recovery journey. We work the Twelve Steps with the guidance of another, more experienced member of the Fellowship, usually our sponsor. We begin to work the Steps the moment we admit that we're out of control in the area of lust. Step work is the heart of the SA Program. As opposed to reading the Steps, believing the Steps, or memorizing the Steps, "*working the Steps*" means taking action. Going to meetings, calling our sponsor, and participating in the Fellowship strengthen our recovery, but unless we are actively working the Steps, we are not working the SA program. *Working the Steps is the SA program of recovery.*

Our self-destructive behaviors and attitudes have been with us for years. We most likely will feel great after having done some writing on a Step. It can take quite a long time to stop the mental hamster wheel and actually sit down and start writing. One technique to kick start writing on a Step is to begin by getting out the materials needed (pen, paper, Step guide, Big Book, White Book). Read the pertinent material and ask God to direct the results. Set a timer for ten minutes, sit down at a table, and start the countdown. Write until the alarm sounds and then decide whether to continue or stop writing. It is both good and important that some work be done for recovery each day. Continuing to write means more progress on the Step. When finished say a prayer of thanks.

### *Slogans*

At times of stress or difficulty, our thoughts can become distorted and confused. When this occurs, it is helpful to have quick catch phrases to help us focus on the solution. Slogans are reminders. They can quickly put our problems or issues into perspective and reduce the unmanageability of a particular situation. Simple by design, slogans can be a powerful way to reconnect to our Program. Slogans are tried and tested. They have lasted because they work. Many have come to us from Alcoholics Anonymous and other Twelve Step Programs.

- Easy Does It
- First Things First
- H.A.L.T. (Hungry, Angry, Lonely, Tired)
- How Important Is It?
- It Works If You Work It
- Keep an Open Mind
- Keep It Simple
- Let Go and Let God
- Let It Begin with Me

- Listen and Learn
- Live and Let Live
- One Day at a Time
- We Claim Progress not Perfection
- This, Too, Shall Pass

As you read through this book and attend meetings, slogans will take on a deeper and more personal meaning.

*Keep coming back!*

### *Daily Recovery Inventory*

Some SA members do a daily renewal call or check-in with another sober member. We call one another every day, usually at the same time, and talk through a script of questions together. One renewal format can be found in our discussion of Step Three. Three other formats appear in *Practical Recovery Tools.* Others are available at meetings or through intergroups. There are also a number of daily phone meetings at which SA members renew their sobriety with others. Some members check in and share on the internet. Contact the SA International Central Office (SAICO), an intergroup, or consult *Essay* for more information.

The daily renewal format, with practice, can be done in five minutes or less. The format keeps us on task, focused on sobriety and on a rigorous working of the Steps. Members report that this connection with another member is a lifeline and can be very useful.

### *Journaling*

One of the most powerful tools for many sexaholics is a journal. We turn to a journal whenever there are strong feelings or dangerous behaviors and write them out. We write out our thoughts and feelings as they come to us; trying to compose artful prose gets us clogged in self-conscious rhetoric. We keep it simple and direct. Often when looking at what we have written, we gain a new perspective on what we were thinking and feeling. We may see what led to our feelings or actions and how these are patterns in our lives. Writing allows us to let go of obsessive thoughts to a piece of paper. Writing also can be shared with a sponsor or SA friend to help get secrets out or to hear another person's response to our inner dialogues.

### *Service**

Service refers to our participation in various activities that contribute to the healthy functioning of the SA Fellowship or help give structure to the SA Program and keep it going. By doing service, we help newcomers find recovery. We freely give back what we've been given, and we enhance our own sobriety in the process. Dr. Bob, one of the founders of Alcoholics Anonymous, put his reasons for doing service in a simple but powerful way:

1. Sense of duty.
2. It is a pleasure.
3. Because in so doing I am paying my debt to the man who took time to pass it on to me.
4. Because every time I do it I take out a little more insurance for myself against a possible slip (*AA* 181).

In the process of doing service, we stay in touch with other members and follow our sponsor's suggestions. We find that, while service does not come naturally at first, it helps us overcome isolation. We feel a sense of usefulness, accomplishment, and inspiration as we see that our actions have a positive impact. We enjoy productive time with other recovering people doing things that carry the message to the suffering sexaholic. Many feel we would have died in our disease without this Fellowship, and it is only through the service of others that our miracle occurred.

- Someone answered the phone to give us information.
- Someone set up the chairs.
- Someone led the meeting.
- Someone came to the meeting week after week, month after month, year after year before we got there.

- Someone led the Newcomer's Meeting.
- Someone talked to us after the meeting.
- Someone brought the literature box.
- Someone minded the treasury.
- Someone maintained Intergroup, regional, and national service structures.
- Someone wrote the books that taught us how to recover.
- Someone organized the Step Workshop, Marathon, or International Convention.
- Someone sponsored our sponsor's sponsor's sponsor.
- Someone ...

There are many kinds of service, from responding to phone calls and attending meetings on the individual level, to serving with others at the group, area, regional, or national and international level. Generally we begin on the individual level and find that, over time, our peace of mind is increased and our sobriety strengthened by broadening our scope of service.

On the individual level, we attend meetings, we keep in touch with other members by making and receiving calls, we sponsor, and we are sponsored. On the group level, we set up chairs, make coffee, or serve as a greeter. We take a service position such as secretary, literature person, treasurer, or meeting chair. We may run orientations for newcomers. We participate in our group's business meetings, which are usually held monthly. We may take notes at these meetings or volunteer to help with an action item that comes up.

We may represent our group at the area Intergroup, which is made up of representatives from the meetings/groups in the area. The Intergroup usually maintains a Post Office Box, fields calls from a phone hotline, and handles outreach to the surrounding community. The Intergroup also acts as a liaison between the groups and the regional and national committees.

We may serve on the Regional Assembly, the General Delegate Assembly (GDA), the Board of Trustees, or various national committees.

*A member of SA shares:*
The more I threw myself into Intergroup work, the less I lusted and the less I fed resentments. I started becoming more aware and mindful of the principles at the foundation of the SA program: honesty, accountability, hopefulness, trust in God's care, acceptance, making restitution for harms caused, and being of use to fellow sufferers. I saw how much the work of the group helped people to find meetings. Workshops, conventions, retreats, and speaker meetings aided group recovery. SA Twelve Step work assisted counselors and clergy to find SA meetings for those in their care. Participation in Intergroup has allowed me to grow in closeness and cooperation with others.

*Working the Traditions*
As Alcoholics Anonymous grew over the first fifteen years, the fellowship found itself challenged with developing basic operating rules. These emerged over a period of years as "The Twelve Traditions—the Long Form" and eventually led to the publication of Twelve Steps and Twelve Traditions. Sexaholics Anonymous adopted the AA Twelve Traditions with only minor changes. At their basic level, the Traditions guide SA in maintaining unity. They show us the role of our leaders as trusted servants. They tell us the requirement for membership in SA and describe our primary purpose. They give us a philosophical foundation for our service structure, for self-support, and for relations with the public.

For most sexaholics with long-term sobriety, the Twelve Traditions mean something more than rules for Twelve Step groups. We study and incorporate the principles of the Twelve Traditions into our personal recovery, as well as applying them for the unity of the Fellowship. We learn that the common welfare of the group as a whole comes before our personal desires. We accept what God provides for us each day, and we serve His purposes ahead of our own. We are thoughtful in our relationships to sexaholics and others in our lives. We become more generous and giving of our time, talents, and resources. We put a priority on sobriety lest we lose everything again. We are cautious about always trying to meet others' expectations. We support ourselves, and we learn to be responsible with our finances. We organize our lives to be useful and accountable. We learn that strong opinions and self-promotion can set us up for possibly deadly drains on our energy. Finally, we remember, as in Step Twelve, that our recovery is rooted in a spiritual experience which we share in common with other sexaholics.

The Twelve Traditions provide a structure for group and individual well-being. They also ensure that Sexaholics Anonymous will be available for the newcomer for as long as there is a need. The Traditions permit sober sexaholics to renew a responsible and useful role in society as a part of, rather than an exception to, the greater whole provided by God as we understand Him. The Twelve Traditions, together with the Twelve Steps, comprise the program of SA.

# *Appendix B*

## *SA Service Positions*

The following lists suggest areas where we can be of service to our groups, intergroups, regions, and committees that serve the fellowship as a whole. More information and complete explanations about service work in SA can be found in the SA Service Manual, which is available from SAICO. If you wish to volunteer for general service, or for more information, call SAICO.

### *Sponsorship*

Local

Long Distance

Prison

### *Service Activities*

Attend meetings.

Share in the solution.

Set-up and/or clean-up.

Provide coffee, tea.

Reach out to newcomers and others who are struggling.

Invite others to get together for a meal or just to talk.

Lead meetings.

Orient newcomers.

Take meetings to prisons and institutions.

Attend workshops, conventions.

Serve on convention committees.

Write and edit for Fellowship publications.

Speak at workshops, conventions.

Organize workshops, conventions.

*Service Positions*

*Group*

Greeter

Secretary

Literature

Sobriety tokens

Treasurer

Audio librarian

Refreshments

Group service representative (GSR) to intergroup

*Intergroup*

Secretary

Literature

Treasurer

Contact information

Public outreach and information

Hospitals and Institutions

Conference/workshop Coordinator

Webmaster

Intergroup representative (IGR) to regional assembly

*Regional*

Chairperson

Vice-chair

Secretary

Treasurer

Delegate to General Delegate Assembly

Alternate delegate



**Appendix B* lists many potential SA service positions.

*International*

General Assembly Delegate
Trustee

*Committees*

Finance
Literature
Correctional Facilities
Hospitals and Institutions
Central Office Management
Nominations
Convention
Internet
Regional Alignment
Legal
Loners
International
Structure

*Special Skills*

Legal
Accounting
Foreign language translation
Technology

# *Appendix C*

## *Some Questions to Consider*

Here is a set of questions to consider as you and your sponsor start working the SA Twelve Step program for recovery from sex addiction.

1. How ready am I to stop my current lustful or sexual behaviors?
2. Do I find that thoughts about sex, romance, or relationships interfere with my daily life?
3. Do I get lost in my head?
4. Do I find that I prefer my fantasies to real life?
5. Do I sexualize the behavior of others?
6. How often do I sexually act out?
7. Do I fantasize, masturbate, or otherwise act out to cover up other feelings?
8. Do I keep violating boundaries that I have set for myself?
9. Do I find myself using the computer for sexual or romantic excitement?
10. Do I prefer my computer activities to the company of real people?
11. Have I lost or damaged relationships because of my behavior?
12. Have I caused myself physical pain or risked my health?
13. Have I experienced remorse, guilt, shame, or depression because of my fantasies or behavior?

## *The Twelve Steps of Sexaholics Anonymous*

1. We admitted we were powerless over lust—that our lives had become unmanageable.
2. Came to believe that a Power greater than ourselves could restore us to sanity.
3. Made a decision to turn our will and our lives over to the care of God *as we understood Him.*
4. Made a searching and fearless moral inventory of ourselves.
5. Admitted to God, to ourselves, and to another human being the exact nature of our wrongs.
6. Were entirely ready to have God remove all these defects of character.
7. Humbly asked Him to remove our shortcomings.
8. Made a list of all persons we had harmed, and became willing to make amends to them all.
9. Made direct amends to such people wherever possible, except when to do so would injure them or others.
10. Continued to take personal inventory and when we were wrong promptly admitted it.
11. Sought through prayer and meditation to improve our conscious contact with God, *as we understood Him*, praying only for knowledge of His will for us and the power to carry that out.
12. Having had a spiritual awakening as the result of these Steps, we tried to carry this message to sexaholics, and to practice these principles in all our affairs.

## *The Twelve Traditions of SA*

1. Our common welfare should come first; personal recovery depends upon SA unity.
2. For our group purpose there is but one ultimate authority—a loving God as He may express Himself in our group conscience. Our leaders are but trusted servants; they do not govern.
3. The only requirement for membership is a desire to stop lusting and become sexually sober.
4. Each group should be autonomous, except in matters affecting other groups or Sexaholics Anonymous as a whole.
5. Each group has but one primary purpose—to carry its message to the sexaholic who still suffers.
6. An SA group ought never endorse, finance, or lend the SA name to any related facility or outside enterprise, lest problems of money, property and prestige divert us from our primary purpose.
7. Every SA group ought to be fully self-supporting, declining outside contributions.
8. Sexaholics Anonymous should remain forever non-professional, but our service centers may employ special workers.
9. SA, as such, ought never be organized; but we may create service boards or committees directly responsible to those they serve.
10. Sexaholics Anonymous has no opinion on outside issues; hence the SA name ought never be drawn into public controversy.
11. Our public relations policy is based on attraction rather than promotion; we need always maintain personal anonymity at the level of press, radio, films, and television.
12. Anonymity is the spiritual foundation of all our Traditions, ever reminding us to place principles before personalities.

## *The Twelve Concepts for SA*

*Concept 1:* Final responsibility and ultimate authority for SA service should always reside in the collective conscience of our whole Fellowship.

*Concept 2:* The leadership of SA, as represented by the General Delegate Assembly and the Board of Trustees, has become for nearly every practical purpose the active voice and the effective conscience of our whole society in its service matters.

*Concept 3:* To ensure effective leadership, we should endow each element of SA's service structure, the General Delegate Assembly and the Board of Trustees and its staffs and Committees with a traditional "Right of Decision."

*Concept 4:* At all responsible levels, we ought to maintain the traditional "Right of Participation," allowing a voting representation in reasonable proportion to the responsibility that each must discharge at that level.

*Concept 5:* Throughout our structure a traditional "Right of Appeal" ought to prevail, so that minority opinion will be heard and personal grievances receive careful consideration.

*Concept 6:* The General Delegate Assembly recognizes that the chief initiative and active responsibility for most service matters should be exercised by the Board of Trustees.

*Concept 7:* The Bylaws of the Board of Trustees are a legal instrument empowering the Board to manage and conduct service matters. The SA service structure documents are not legal documents. They rely on tradition and the SA purse for final effectiveness.

*Concept 8:* The Trustees are the principal administrators of overall policy and finance.

*Concept 9:* Good service leadership at all levels is indispensable for our future functioning and safety.

*Concept 10:* Every service responsibility should be matched by an equal service authority, with scope of such authority well defined.

*Concept 11:* The Trustees should always have the assistance of the best possible committees, staffs and consultants. Composition, qualifications, induction procedures, rights and duties will always be matters of serious concern.

*Concept 12:* The General Delegate Assembly and the Board of Trustees shall observe the spirit of SA tradition, taking care that it never becomes the seat of perilous wealth or power, that sufficient operating funds, plus an ample reserve, be its prudent financial principle, that it place none of its members in a position of unqualified authority over others; that it reach all important decisions by discussion, vote and whenever possible by substantial unanimity; that its actions never be personally punitive nor an incitement to public controversy; that it never perform acts of government; and that like the Fellowship it serves, it will always remain democratic in thought and action.

SA, as such, would never have an organization in the sense of a "government" that could issue directives by committee or Board to individuals or groups within the fellowship. Our committees and Board could only provide services and we've tried to organize them to function effectively. But SA has no government in the political sense.*

*"The Co-Founders of Alcoholics Anonymous (Biographical sketches their last major talks)," Pg 25

The Twelve Concepts for SA approved by the General Delegate Assembly, January 2004

## *Sexaholics Anonymous Statement of Principle*

We have a solution. We don't claim it's for everybody, but for us, it works. If you identify with us and think you may share our problem, we'd like to share our solution with you (*Sexaholics Anonymous*, last sentence, page 2).

In defining sobriety, we do not speak for those outside Sexaholics Anonymous. We can only speak for ourselves. Thus, for the married sexaholic, sexual sobriety means having no form of sex with self or with persons other than the spouse. In SA's sobriety definition, the term "spouse" refers to one's partner in a marriage between a man and a woman. For the unmarried sexaholic, sexual sobriety means freedom from sex of any kind. And for all of us, single and married alike, sexual sobriety also includes progressive victory over lust (Sexaholics Anonymous, 191-192).

The only requirement for SA membership is a desire to stop lusting and become sexually sober according to the SA sobriety definition.

Any two or more sexaholics gathered together for SA sobriety according to the SA sobriety definition may call themselves an SA group.

Meetings that do not adhere to and follow Sexaholics Anonymous' sobriety statement as set forth in the foregoing Statement of Principle adopted by the General Delegate Assembly in 2010 are not SA meetings and shall not call themselves SA meetings.

*Addendum to the Statement of Principle passed by the General Delegate Assembly on July 8, 2016. Moved to publish the addendum to the Statement of Principle in all SAICO literature, Essay, SA.org home page, SA Service Manual, and through the SA service structure.*

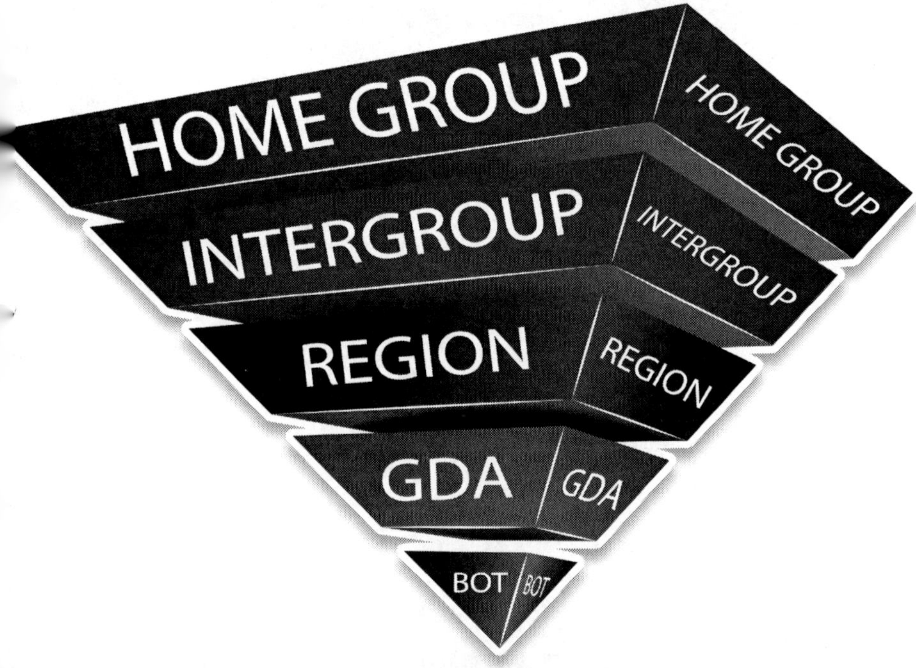


***Home Group***
Our home group is where we discover sobriety and recovery. The home group is also where we first learn to give back to others through service.

***Intergroup***
The Intergroup is composed of Group Service Representatives (GSR's) from all the meetings in a designated area. The Intergroup should seek both the knowledge of God's will for the Fellowship and the power to carry it out.

***Region***
Just as groups in a designated area come together in an Intergroup to serve their area, Intergroups come together to serve their Region on the National and International level. The Region is composed of Intergroup Representatives (IGR's). The Region elects Delegates to the General Delegate Assembly (GDA).

***General Delegate Assembly***
The General Delegate Assembly (GDA) provides policy guidelines for the Fellowship as a whole. The GDA is the active voice and effective conscience of the Fellowship. The GDA also nominates, interviews and elects members of the Board of Trustees.

***Board of Trustees***
The Board of Trustees oversees *Essay* and SAICO. The Board is responsible for ensuring that SAICO is compliant with all laws and regulations governing non-profit organizations. The Trustees take direction from and are answerable to the General Delegate Assembly.

I am responsible.
When anyone, anywhere
reaches out for help,
I want the hand of SA
always to be there.
And for that:
I am responsible.